How  Spot a Liar

How to Be More Effective at Reading People's Body Language

(A Practical Guide to Speed Read People, Decipher Body Language, Detect Deception and Get to the Truth)

Jack Garner

Published By **Ryan Princeton**

Jack Garner

All Rights Reserved

How to Spot a Liar: How to Be More Effective at Reading People's Body Language (A Practical Guide to Speed Read People, Decipher Body Language, Detect Deception and Get to the Truth)

ISBN 978-1-998901-52-4

No part of this guidebook shall be reproduced in any form without permission in writing from the publisher except in the case of brief quotations embodied in critical articles or reviews.

Legal & Disclaimer

The information contained in this ebook is not designed to replace or take the place of any form of medicine or professional medical advice. The information in this ebook has been provided for educational & entertainment purposes only.

The information contained in this book has been compiled from sources deemed reliable, and it is accurate to the best of the Author's knowledge; however, the Author cannot guarantee its accuracy and validity and cannot be held liable for any errors or omissions. Changes are periodically made to this book. You must consult your doctor or get professional medical advice before using any of the suggested remedies, techniques, or information in this book.

Upon using the information contained in this book, you agree to hold harmless the Author from and against any damages, costs, and expenses, including any legal fees potentially resulting from the application of any of the information provided by this guide. This disclaimer applies to any damages or injury caused by the use and application, whether directly or indirectly, of any advice or information presented, whether for breach of contract, tort, negligence, personal injury, criminal intent, or under any other cause of action.

You agree to accept all risks of using the information presented inside this book. You need to consult a professional medical practitioner in order to ensure you are both able and healthy enough to participate in this program.

Table Of Contents

Chapter 1: The Fallacy of the Polygraph Machine

Polygraph machines, often called the "lie detector" has a prominent place within popular culture. It's often featured as a part of police FBI as well as CIA movies and is even utilized to create comic effects in films like Meet the Fockers. It is believed that the machine is able to precisely determine if the people in question are lying. It isn't.

The reality is that polygraph machines are susceptible to being fooled, with false and misleading results. typical.

It's not uncommon for applicants to pass an examination to be able to get Federal government or security job opportunities. Many police departments utilize them for interviews of prospective candidates, and so does those from the CIA along with the FBI. If these highly regarded government agencies employ them, they should be reliable, right?

But not so fast. If a lie detector could accurately detect lies would it not serve as a the point that we no longer needed legal courts? All we'd need be able to do is to hook someone onto a machine that detects lies and find out if they've committed the offense. If they do, ask them to admit it and , if the lie detector proves that they're lying, they're declared guilty and sent to the jail.

It would be nice if things were this easy. Polygraph machines are so unreliable that the results usually aren't legally admissible in the courtroom. They are more of an effective scare tactic rather than an effective method to assess whether or not someone is lying. Most often, people hooked to the polygraph machine think that they'll be snared if they are lying, and so they open up and confess when confronted with probing questions about the offenses they're suspected of. Test results from the lie detection test can't be used in court however, the confessions that are elicited from the test subjects are admissible.

The scientific basis behind these machines is more an ounce uncertain. Many scientists who aren't any way connected to the industry of lie detection will claim that lies detection can be more like a pseudoscience, rather than the truth.

The control question is the most popular type of lie detection used currently. It is based on the baseline measurements of a variety of physiological indicators and then compares it with the results when a individual is asked questions, which could be lying. This is a bit more complex as I'm hoping to make seem however the basic idea is that if two measurements differ significantly and the result is that the second question will be deemed to be a lie.

The test is designed to measure anxiety as evident by an increase in breathing rate, heart rate as well as blood pressure. The issue is that the test can't distinguish the normal stress from that that is caused by lying. If the subject is anxious during the interview the results could vary significantly even when they are lying. External factors can trigger variations in breathing rate, heart rate as well as blood pressure. It's possible for a question to make someone anxious or anxious, regardless whether they're telling the truth.

It's believed that up to 15% of the results that are positive for lying can be false positives. This is a great deal of uncertainty regarding the reliability in the results. If you take into account that the test is conducted as part of internal investigations within high-security firms and by even the government itself, it raises the question of how many employees have been dismissed due to fake positive test results.

While false positives can be an issue as well, false negatives are also a common occurrence in test results in the amount around 1 in every 10 individuals tested. You've now got an average of in the region of 10-30 percent of people who are examined showing false results. It's no wonder that polygraph test results typically aren't admissible in court. It's quite surprising that they're being employed at all considering the fact that they're not accurate.

Let's suppose that false results are on the lower end on the scale, producing just 10% of results being incorrect. That's a total of 10 out of 100 people examined, with less than exact results. When you look at it from a purely statistical perspective the number doesn't sound at all. For all we know 90% of the people who were tested showed accurate results. Let's examine the implications.

These tests are run to The CIA as well as the FBI to determine if any spying activities have taken place. It is possible to find one out of the ten people who are being investigated or questioned being able to conceal the truth and still get away with it and being falsely accused doing something they did not do. This is a minimum of one hundred out of every thousand test subjects that are at risk of losing their jobs due to reasons that aren't legitimate, other than the fact that they're not able to pass a test that has been proven repeatedly to be in error and insufficient. Not to mention those spies who haven't been found guilty.

Do you need more proof? You need to look no further than a 1983 study from the Congressional Office of Technology Assessment (OTA) that was titled "Scientific validity of polygraph testing." The report suggests that as 50 innocent persons could be found guilty for every one who is actually innocent. Even with 99 percent accuracy rate -- a one that's undisputed the polygraph test's validity, ten innocent individuals are found guilty for each person who is actually guilty.

It's a huge number of people being charged with false accusations for each person who is really in fact guilty. It's more than bizarre that a test that is used to find truth is infamous for generating false results.

Can a Person Beat the Polygraph Machine?

If you inquire about the individuals who conduct the tests to answer the questions, they will give you an emphatic "NO." They'll tell you that an experienced polygraph reader can detect when someone is lying, no matter what techniques they employ to confuse the results. If you inquire about the polygraph detractor to explain the tests, they'll say they can be beat using a variety of methods that can make it impossible to discern whether a person is lying.

Like the most hotly debated topics The answer is between. Anyone who isn't equipped with understanding of the workings of the polygraph test isn't likely to be capable of stepping into an examination and beat the machine. However those who are proficient in beating the polygraph test will employ several countermeasures that create inaccurate or inaccessible results.

Physical countermeasures are able to trigger an emotional responses from our bodies. This physical reaction can outweigh the body's emotional reaction to lying. Individuals who chew their tongues or lips, press their toes against the thumbtack of their shoes, or push the nails of their hands or fingers could trigger physiological reactions that are comparable to the responses that their body releases when they false story.

They can deceive the machine by using physical countermeasures in the control question phase , when they're asked questions they're clearly required to answer all the facts about. If they're confronted with a question they'll be lying about, they perform the same action inducing the same reaction from their body. Expertly trained subjects may confuse test results until it's difficult to discern the distinction between lies and truth.

Add this to the capacity of some people to separate them from what they tell and you'll be able to beat the machine consistently. Expertly trained subjects can boost their responses to controlled questions and detach themselves from the pertinent questions. This is why polygraphs are ineffective for the most part in secure settings where the subjects will have been trained on how to defeat the machine.

These two techniques could be detected by a competent examiner. While an examiner may not be able tell whether or not the individual is lying, he might be able to discern if the suspect is manipulating the system. There ishowever another countermeasure that is more difficult to identify.

9

Tranquilizing drugs that reduce the body's reaction to lying aren't so difficult to identify. These drugs produce similar results to tests regardless of whether the subject is truthful or lying. The test results being dismissed as not conclusive.

Chapter 2: Becoming a Human Lie Detector

Although polygraph tests are wildly ineffective, you can be an actual human lie detector that is more effective than the devices currently in use. To be able to do this successfully you must be able to discern the words someone else is saying to you using their body and making sure it is in line with the words coming out of their mouth.

An individual's actions, accent on facial expressions, speech cadence eyes, and the way they behave during conversation can be used to determine whether or not the person is speaking the truth. If you look at them in conjunction with the words spoken you will be able to recognize the lies.

There are several common signs to be looking for to determine if an individual is lying. When you are aware of these signs and indicators, you'll be able to tell the signs that you've been lied to. It's your decision whether you'd like to expose the person who is lying as an obscene fraud. Beware, the majority of people will not consider being able to discern the body language of a person as a legitimate reason for you to know they're lying. We'll go over ways to identify an liar in the next chapter.

In order to be a successful person who can detect lies, you'll have to discern a person's identity from top to the bottom. Beginning with your feet and work your way towards the head and head, the process of reading a lie becomes increasingly complicated. Let's start with the feet , and take the simple stuff out firstbefore we move on to the more difficult stuff, and finish by reading facial expressions or eye movements.

When analyzing body language, you must be looking for a set of signs that suggest the person is lying. A couple of these indicators alone do not necessarily mean that a person is lying. Combining these indicators generally will. Instead of looking for one indicator or taking move, look for "sentences" that indicate the lie. Look at the person's actions behavior and words in a holistic way, not as a series of isolated actions that don't connect to one another.

Chapter 3: The Feet, Legs and Knees

The legs and feet are among the most difficult parts of the body that can be read when it comes to lying because the majority of people don't have a sense about what the feet or legs are doing when they're talking. Arm and hand movements are controlled during conversations especially by a master lying liar trying to appear sincere. The feet and legs usually aren't as well controlled.

Our feet expose a lot about us. They show what we think towards the individual we're speaking to as well as the extent to which we're attracted sexually to the person we're talking to and how we feel about ourselves in general. Our feet can show our true feelings since they're the part of our body which is farthest to our minds. It's easy to forget about the activities of our feet rather we focus at our faces and hands.

To comprehend the leg and foot movements and directions It is important to know the things we utilize our feet and legs for most. The legs and feet move us towards things we enjoy and want, while avoiding things we don't want. Pay focus on what a person is doing using their feet and legs because it is the part of the body where a person is most likely not to control consciously while speaking.

We are wired move instinctively towards food sources and to flee from danger. This has been instilled into us since the dawn of the human race. It's normal for our knees, feet and legs to be pointed in the direction that they'd like to travel. If someone is feeling uncomfortable because of lying down on their feet, legs and knees could be a sign of weakness. If you're talking with someone and their feet are pointed at the door, it is an indication that it's time to end the conversation. The person you're talking with is looking to leave no matter what words they're using using their mouth.

The legs and feet pointed at the out of the way towards you or out of your sight indicates that the person you're talking to prefers to be elsewhere. This could be due to being bored or they're not comfortable with the subject at hand. You should be aware of the signs that they are shifting their feet and legs away from you if you suspect that they are lying.

It is common sense to look for a sudden foot movement, like tapping your feet against the desk or on the ground, when trying to discern whether the person you are talking to is lying. This type of movement is believed to signify that a person is unsure of what they are discussing and could be lying. This is a generalization and doesn't provide a reliable indicator of the truthfulness.

To read the person's feet to discern whether they're lying and how they move, observe them when they're talking to each other in normal conversation. Pay attention to how their feet move and try to determine a base to what their typical foot movements are while they're talking and lying. This will allow you to observe sudden, unusual shifts in how the feet move.

Naturally anxious people tend to move their feet or move their feet around every day. It's not just a matter of when they're making up stories. Actually, those who are prone to tapping their feet and fidgeting when they are lying tend to stop tapping their feet while lying in a conscious effort to ward off this nervous response. If you're merely checking for foot movements that are rapid it is possible to interpret the foot tapping of a person who is nervous as an indication of lying and will interpret the stop of tapping as a sign that the person is who is lying.

If someone fidgets and taps their feet often in normal conversation, and then suddenly stop all motion and then stops all motion, it's a sign they're lying. However it is if one's feet remain stationary most of the time, and then suddenly they begin to move rapidly which is also a sign the lie is in the air (pun not intended).

There are also differentiating factors between genders. Men are more likely to exhibit increased feet movement when they are stressed and women tend to be less active with their feet. If you notice a man's foot movements increase or a woman's foot movements slows down during a conversation The person could be lying.

A person who sits down and is honest is more likely to keep their legs open and their backs to the other direction. This is true more so for women than men as a majority of Western women are taught that it's a sign of respect to have their legs crossed rather than wide.

For women, where their legs are pointed can be more revealing. If their feet or legs are pointed toward you it signifies that they don't want to be there or fearful and aren't keen on the conversation to go on. This could simply mean they're bored in tears, this could be an indication that they're in a state of discomfort because they're lying.

When someone has the legs cross, notice at the place where the knee of the highest leg is facing. In the event that the knee's pointed towards the person they're speaking to, it means that they are attracted by the person they're talking to and are less likely to tell an untruth. The farther away from the knee that it is pointed towards, the more likely the person is lying. A knee that points towards an exit indicates that the person is desperate to get out of the way.

Check out how tightly the legs of the person are crossed. The tightness of the legs indicates the feeling of defensiveness. Someone is trying to shield themselves from you.

Look out for sudden changes in your posture if you suspect that someone may be lying. If someone is lying with their legs open or partially open, and then suddenly crosses their legs could be secretly sealing themselves in with their feet by closing them before or during a lying confession.

Be aware that the more time a person sits and the longer they'll change positions in order to remain at a comfortable position. If a person is sitting for longer than 20-30 minutes might change the position of their legs due to their legs being uncomfortable and they're shifting towards a more comfortable posture.

If you're in the situation where you believe that someone might lie towards you, try to position yourself in a spot in which you can observe the things they're doing with their arms, legs and feet. In the event that the person who you're speaking to is sitting behind a large desk that hinders your view of lower portion of their bodies, attempt to put your body in the room in a way that you are able to see part of what they're doing with their feet and legs. If the person tries to change their position so that it is impossible to see their feet or legs they may be making an attempt to obscure the most visible portion of their body away from you.

When you're standing people, be aware of the posture of their feet. A broad stance suggests confidence and a person who feels that they are in charge of their situation. The closer they are to their feetthe more secure they feel. If their feet are pointed toward the opposite person who they're speaking to, it's a sign that they'd like to quit the conversation, often due to boredom, or because they're unhappy with the direction in which the conversation is heading.

Check the distance between yourself with the individual you're talking with. If the person veers off or moves to a more remote location in conversation, this could indicate that a lie is coming. The person is trying to create some distance between themselves and you due to lying. This makes them feel uncomfortable, and they're concerned you'll be able tell whether they're lying if they remain near.

When you're watching someone's body language it's easy to become lost in trying to understand their facial expressions, arm and hand motions. Foot movements and leg movements are frequently left out. Do not make this mistake because the legs and feet are more transparent as well as less likely to be manipulated.

Chapter 4: The Hips Don't Lie

This article is likely to be brief however, it's imperative to pay attention to the information you read. The hips are just as transparent as the feet as well as knees and feet in discerning the lies.

There are some things to be aware of in regards to hips. Someone who is confident and strong will push their hips forward, usually when they lean back. This can indicate confidence or sexual attraction from the person who is pushing their legs forward. It's not the typical stance one who's engaged in lying would take. They're often worried about getting caught lying and tend to pull their hips back.

Someone who is lying may want to remove their hips out of their natural instinct. When you lie, your body will to react to what it sees as the possibility of danger by removing the genitals and shielding them.

Be aware of the position of the hands in relation the hips. Hands on hips is an aggressive posture that is usually avoided by people who are in the middle of telling a lie and being serene. If there is a dispute the odds are stacked against you and the hands on the hips could be a sign that someone is lying and will argue about it. Be aware of a person's hands to move defensively towards their sexual organs. Someone who is prone to cover their genitals might be worried about something.

Similar to the feet and legs The direction that the hips point will reveal the true intentions of the individual. If your hips face you is probably in conversation and likely to lie. If someone suddenly shifts their hips towards the door feels uncomfortable and would like to go home.

If it's about hips and lies, this is it. They'll either be out or in either facing your face or not. All you need is an instant glance to see what your hips tell you.

Chapter 5: The Torso

The torso is comprised of the stomach chest, back, and shoulders. In the event of detecting lying, the upper section of the torso can be more significant than the lower part. The stomach doesn't play a role in determining who is lying.

The upper body in contrast emits a series of easy-to-read signals that indicate if someone is lying. We've all heard of "giving your shoulder a cold." If you're speaking to someone and observe their body is swaying to the point that their chest isn't facing you, then you're suffering from"the "cold shoulder." This is a sign of the desire to not engage in conversation. If someone entirely around in the direction of your conversation, then they're trying to block your communication with them generally since the topic is unsettling for them or has made them uncomfortable.

The shoulders that are rolled or hunched is another indication that a person feels uncomfortable, which could be because they lie. It indicates that the person feels less important than you and feels submissive. If you suspect that they're lying and you observe the person hunch or roll the shoulders of their back, this might be a good idea to gently press them to try to get them to give in. You should also look for them to rub or touch their chest. This is another indication of tension or stress.

Pay attention to the movement of the chest of the individual to determine whether their breathing rate rises or decreases. Breathing that is rapid or intense indicates an increased emotional state. It could indicate nervousness or fear.

If someone is lying, they could raise their shoulders or reduce their heads. This is a natural attempt to safeguard the neck from injury. Although the chance of a physical attack typically negligible but when the body's instincts take over as a response to fear, it isn't able to distinguish between mental and physical attacks. The brain detects danger and immediately responds to it by defending vulnerable zones.

Look out for an unusually rigid body. If someone's upper body movements seem like they are manipulated or mechanical, then they could be trying to block their natural movements to hide an untruth.

Find shoulder shrugs that substitute for spoken words. Shrugs instead of a reply could indicate that someone isn't willing to speak in fear of being caught out in a lie. People tend to shrug when they're feeling uncomfortable, and they don't even realize the fact that they've done it.

An incomplete shrug could be more likely suggest a lie than an entire shrug. A real shrug that means "I I don't have any idea" is most likely to be a full shrug of shoulders, with both shoulders rising to fall in unison. Shrugs in which one shoulder is higher than another or where both of them are stopped halfway is a fake one that is used to conceal deceit.

Chapter 6: The Arms and Hands

The hands and arms are among the most active parts in the body in conversations. Some movements of hands and arms are controlled, while other occur without the person who is doing them conscious of what they're doing.

The first thing you should observe in regards to the hands and arms is the place they're placed. A folded chest with arms signify a defensive posture. A person protects vital organs by creating the appearance of a barrier that protects their chest. These "barriers" suggest a person who is anxious about something and is looking to shut themselves off.

The same is true to those who cover his or her genitals using hands. It is also a way to shield a delicate area and can be a sign of anxiety or anxiety.

Be aware of less obvious arm barriers that are placed behind you by the one you think of lying. Someone who is holding a book, or purse close to their chest can create an obstacle. It's the same for someone who extends across their body using one arm to hold a beverage at the table.

Someone who holds his hands in front of their backs is confident. This is a common position held by people who are in a position who are in a position of authority, such as officials of the law or royals. They take on this role because they feel powerful enough that they believe they are able to expose themselves to attack without fear. The person who takes such a position feels confident and confident. They're either honest or they're not worried about being and caught up in the lies they're telling.

The hands are the area of the body with majority of nerve endings that connect to brain. They're also the area of the body that is most likely to display symptoms of internal stress and frustration. Be aware of nervous reactions in hands. A swaying of the legs or arms, securing the other limb in tight gripping an object or clothes is a sign of tension.

Another sign to look out for using your hands is excessive scratching, tapping or scratching. Naturally anxious people can be prone to this behavior all the time. Pay attention to these individuals' actions and accelerate or slow their behavior in the event that you suspect they are lying.

An open display of the inner arms, palms facing upwards is an act of sincerity. Salespeople and speakers have been trained to use this method to benefit themselves Be aware that things might not be as simple as it appears with regards to this gesture. If you're talking with someone who's not received professional training, it could suggest sincerity. Be sure to consider this in relation to the others in their body language.

Do not confuse a display of palms as a palms down gesture. Hands down gestures indicate the dominance. If palms are employed to strike an unflat surface, such as a table, the goal is to make the words appear to be truthful. It is possible to emphasise a point by lying in order in order to make it appear more authentic.

The clenched fists of a person symbolize either fear or anger. Someone is clenching their fists due to either either to stop the anger they're trying keep from releasing or because they're afraid of striking the thing. If you're in a conversation with someone and they hold their hands in a fist, check them out!

Chapter 7: The Head and Neck

The neck and the head are the part of our body that are closest to our brain. Our face, as well as our hands and arms are the body parts that body that we are most likely to notice when we're talking. We alter our neck and head positions along by using our hands and arms to show our emotions that we believe we ought to display.

The book will be divided into several sections. The first one will focus on the neck and head region in general. Following that we'll finish by focusing on facial expressions and eye movements.

The Head and Neck

The neck and the head as a whole must be inspected for any small "tells" that indicate the person is lying. The obvious head and neck movements are not necessarily intentional and could reveal the real purpose behind what a person is thinking or saying. The more subtle movements that you must be on the lookout for.

The first sign is a subtle nod or head shake during your conversation or when the person you're talking to is talking. It is important to look for the subtle head nod or shake. Head movements that are large tend to be deliberate and can be seen as an attempt to express a desire to be in agreement or disagreement. The smallest movements are not intentional and reveal the person's real thoughts.

Here's a list of most likely meanings for head shakes and nods:

A nod in the obvious when the person is speaking. An attempt to persuade you to believe the words they're using.

A nod in the midst of talking. An attempt to indicate that you are in agreement with you.

A subtle nod when the person is speaking. This indicates that the person accepts the message on a subconscious level.

Nod in a subdued way while you're speaking. It indicates that the person is in agreement with the message on a subconscious level.

A noticeable head shake when the person is speaking. A deliberate attempt to indicate disagreement with what the subject is discussing.

A noticeable head shake when you're talking. The person you're talking with does not agree with what you're saying , and would like to express that.

* Subtle head shakes when the subject is speaking. It is important to take it in the context of. It could indicate an internal conflict which the individual is not happy with the words they are uttering from their mouths.

"Subtle head shakes while you're speaking. The person isn't happy with the way you're speaking However, they're not trying to tell you.

Pay attention to the neck and the Adam's apple. A lot of swallowing or movement of the Adam's Apple indicates discomfort, and could be a sign of the possibility of a lie.

The clearing of the throat could indicate that the subject would like to express their opinion but is not letting the words in. The clear throat is a way to express their frustration. The excessive clearing of the throat could be an attempt to fool.

Someone who raises their arms and puts a single hand on their neck or head, or raises their head and play with their back ear is feeling internal tension. This is usually an indication of negative emotions. If you're asking someone questions it's a sign someone is trying to hide something. This is a great moment to ask for more details. If the person is able to put both hands on their heads it's a sign of strength. They're in a good mood and aren't concerned about what's happening.

Look for hand movements that are quick towards the back of the neck or the head in the course of a conversation. I've observed that greater force in the hand movements is, the more likely the person may be hiding something or denying details.

The Eyes and Eye Movements

Eye movements are a part of the face that most people aren't conscious of. This is why it's crucial to pay attention at the eyes.

The pupils display our real emotions in relation to our faces. Positive emotions cause pupils to dilate, whereas the negative emotions cause them to constrict. A majority of people have little to none ability to control the dilation in their pupils therefore, it is important to keep an check on the pupils.

The eyelids' position can be used to determine the way a person is feeling. If someone is calm, they is likely to have more of the upper eyelid that covers their eyes, whereas a person who is stressed will have less of the lower eyelid. If they feel uncomfortable, they might reduce the distance between their eyes. If someone you're talking with suddenly is able to narrow their eyes and is unsure of what they're going to say the next time.

Gaze avoidance is when someone abruptly shifts their head away from eye contact with you when they are talking. This is more frequent among teenagers and children than adults. The majority of them are insecure until they do not want to look at each other. For children younger than this, it is an act of shame.

There has been a lot made of eye contact, relating to lying. Certain books advise to look for excessive eye contact. Other books advise to be on the lookout for too much eye contact. It's my experience that it's best to establish an established baseline in regards to eye contact, and then observe for any signs that the person may depart from that baseline. If a person is consistently making eye contact in normal conversations Then, they break contact and does not gaze at you it's likely that they're doing something that makes them feel guilty.

For someone who seldom engages in eye contact during an interaction, the opposite happens. If someone who isn't making eye contact, but suddenly looks at you with eyes when talking about something is trying to offer you a false claim of items.

When a person is lying down, they lying position is likely to look downwards at their floor and avoid any eye contact. This downward glance may or might not be followed by a forward tilt of the head. This means that all of the face is pointing towards the floor. If someone is telling the truth, they're most likely to be looking at exactly the same height as you do and be able to stare at you. A lying person won't be tempted to engage in eye contact because they fear the risk of exposing themselves.

Eye contact is normal and lasts about three to four seconds. Anything more than that could suggest an attempt to draw you into believing some untruth.

There are two very famous cases where individuals who later proved to be lying , exhibited an empathetic look when they were engaged in lying. If you're interested, take a look at Richard Nixon's "I am not a crook" as well as Bill Clinton's "I didn't have sexual relationships with that woman" appeal for all American citizens on Youtube.

Rapid blinking indicates distress. An increased rate of blinking or fluttering the eyelids is observed in some people each when they lie. Because this response is linked with the nervous system's central nerves, it's nearly impossible to disguise it.

Do not mistake fast blinking as eyelid bats, which is a regular occurrence in courtship with the other sex.

The way a person's eyes are directed while answering a question can give an indication of whether they are speaking honestly or not. If someone is looking to the left when answering a question could be trying to create a story they are telling in their head. If someone is looking to the right may be recalling something, and then pulling it out of their memory. Switch these directions to people who are left-handed.

Facial Expressions and Emotions

Face expressions are the way into the heart. They're the primary way that we communicate our feelings and emotions to other people. Be aware that facial expressions can be used by professional lying liars to communicate sincerity and confidence.

Consider facial expressions in relation in relation to what the body language the subject is speaking. In the event that the facial expression displayed on display isn't in line with the facial expressions in the display, the subject will likely be trying to to convince you that they're lying.

Similar to the pupils of our eyes, our facial muscles tend to get tighter and narrow when we're feeling anxious or stressed. Look for lips that are pursed or eyes that are closed partially and an overall look of tension that suggests that muscles of the face are tightening. Lips that are pursed can be an indication of someone who is not sharing important information. If you ask someone directly an inquiry when they purse their lips but do not acknowledge that they know There's a good possibility that they have more information than they're willing to admit.

In the event that you question someone what is wrong and they inform that

42

everything is fine with their mouths shut, everything is not right. They're hiding something, which could be released with more pushing. The lips tightly closed are an unconscious attempt to keep the contents.

A jaw that is clenched and grinds teeth indicate anger or frustration. Take care not to press a person with these signs as they could be on edge of losing control. Someone who is lying might show signs of anger when you ask them questions about what they are lying about.

Blushing or flushing is a different thing we have do about. The sudden redness of cheeks could be caused through shame, embarrassment or anger.

Smiles are among the most fake facial expressions available. A forced smile is only made up of lips, whereas an authentic smile is one that involves the whole face. A genuine smile typically reveals the crow's feet visible around one of the eye's corners.

A fake smile can be concealing something. A genuine smile is not a burden for the imagination. You can tell that the person who is happy both inside and outside.

Someone who is awed by the direction in which a conversation is taking may take a break for a moment , then stand in a position with their mouth wide. This shows the person is in shock. The more the mouth expands and the jaw drops the more amazed they appear. When accompanied by wide, open eyes, fear could be the dominant emotion.

Be aware of inappropriate display of emotion, or the absence of emotion when it is appropriate. If you make a small claim and they explode in anger, blaming anything, you've revealed a possible lie. In the same vein If you're accusing someone of something such as infidelity, and there's very little or no emotional reaction then there's a high likelihood an untruth will soon be revealed. The emotions that aren't suitable to the circumstances could indicate that something is happening in the background.

A quick gesture of the tongue between closed lips signifies frustration or displeasure. If you're adamant about your opinion and you observe them sticking their tongue in front of their mouth, it's a high chance that they don't agree with your opinion. The gesture of the tongue with the lips is usually a sign of negative feelings.

The next thing to consider is something the majority of people don't think of as deceit that is the smile. If you're in the middle of a conversation, and the person with whom you're conversing is suddenly all yawning This could be a sign that the person doesn't agree with you. It could also indicate that you're boring. However, it's a sign that you need to take a deeper look. You can ask a few queries to find out if they provoke some response.

When speaking to children, be aware of the children to reach up or cover their mouths. This is a clear indicator that they're not being honest. As we get older the hand placed over the mouth gets less obvious. Instead of placing our hands over our mouths and then leaving it there, we raise our hand and lightly touch our mouths. Check for any erupting mouth touch. People will instinctively make contact with their mouths but stop short of touching their mouths and then put their hands on the floor.

If someone is engaged in lying they'll be more prone to displaying facial expressions as well as expressions of emotion are delayed longer than in normal. They'll speak, and then exhibit the emotion associated with what they've said. The emotion may appear exaggerated, and it will likely end abruptly, instead of fading away as normal emotions do. If someone is lying about something is likely to shut down their emotions and back on in an effort to convince you that they're sincere. A person who is honest doesn't have to struggle to control their emotions.

Verbal Clues You're Being Lied To

I am aware that this book is mostly about body language, but in order to be a true detector of lies, one need be capable of recognizing visual cues and also read the body language of a person. telling you.

They are more likely to avoid telling the truth about something, rather choosing to play the game. If you ask an open-ended question and they fail to respond to the question, odds are that they're trying not to risk being a lie. Try to force them to give you an answer , and then watch their body language to find additional indications that they're lying. A person who is honest does not have anything to hide and will often not answer directly to a question.

Watch for the person to repeat the question back to you. When you inquire "Did you steal cash from my account?" And they reply "No I didn't take the money from in your wallet" you're likely to find you've identified the person who stole your money. If someone is lying, they is likely to repeat the words you're using to emphasize it.

In the event that you inquire about something that is expected to get a straight answer and get a lengthy response that contains details that you didn't request It's likely that the person who answers you is lying. A lie-teller will try to give as much detail as they can. In the last resort, they'll usually name individuals who can prove they're lying. This is usually going to be trusted friends that who they can count on to verify their claim. Beware of this strategy. The most reputable lying liars are able to work their alibis out before they even begin especially in the case of sensitive topics.

Pay attention to the rhythm of the person you suspect to be lying. Do they typically talk in a jolly manner? Look for signs that the subject is trying to change their style of speaking. Also , pay attention to the emphasis being placed on words that isn't appropriate to focus on. They are trying to force words from their mouths . They don't always know how to emphasis what they're saying.

Take note of the person you are talking to is in the direction of offensive or defensive. If someone is lying, they is likely to be defensive. They'll feel that they're being targeted and might be hesitant to answer any questions. It's not unusual for the guilty party to try to shift the blame onto the victim.

An innocent person will not be defensive. Instead, they'll take the offensive. They might show expressions of anger over being accused of lying However, they'll try everything to show you that they aren't lying. Instead of refusing to answer questions they'll open up to answering your questions in a sincere effort to get their reputation back.

5 Questions To Ask Yourself If You Think You're Being Lied To

This list of questions is a list of questions to consider asking yourself when you suspect you're being deceived. This list can help develop your lie-detecting abilities into a fine art.

1.) What really matters it matters if it's a lie?

This should be the very first inquiry you make each time you begin to notice the signs that of a lie being presented. The majority of the time you can answer with a clear No. If it's not a problem and doesn't harm anyone there's no need to spend time on it.

When you've mastered your craft enough, you'll be amazed by how many times people are lying. Many people lie frequently Some lie only on occasion, while certain people lie when it's convenient for their needs. The question of whether it actually is important allows you to eliminate the irrelevant lies. You'll recognize that the person lies, but it doesn't have to be taken action on.

2.) How many signs are there?

Check out the amount of signs and see how many are in the area. If the person is presenting numerous indicators or the signs are very strong, you're witnessing the act of deceit. When you've decided you've been duped then it's time to move and ask the following question.

When I first began when I first started, I would use an organized approach. I began with my feet and moved to the upper part of the body while trying to find body language signals. After I had scanned the individual's body for indications of lying I then began to observe how they spoke.

Since I'm a skilled lie detector, I'm able quickly scan people to find signs of lying and listen to what they're saying , and then tearing the pieces apart in my mind. I've practiced it so many times that it's a natural thing to me. It takes time and time, but with time, you'll be able to train yourself to be alert and on the lookout for danger.

3.) What am I likely to gain or lose in the event that I expose this lie?

Sometimes, it's better to let a massive lie go. There's no way to benefit from disclosing that your boss has been lying on their daily accounts. What you'll do is prove to your boss that you aren't taken seriously and discredit yourself in the organization.

However the time to expose an untruth can be extremely beneficial to you. It's your decision to decide on when and when not expose an untruth in the eyes of the entire world.

4.) Have I sufficient evidence to disprove the truth at the moment?

Before you call foul, take a examine the evidence in the case against someone you're trying to expose. Do you have evidence and witnesses to support it or will it just be your words against the truth? If it's the latter's word against yours what is chances that those whom you're trying to expose will believe it? Do the person you're trying to expose already have a history of this type of behavior or will it be shocking? The more shocking it is and the more unlikely people will believe it when you don't provide them with evidence.

5) Do I have my escape route?

People who are constantly lying are often clever people. They've devoted their lives to lying and have perfected the art form. If you encounter such a person you'll have to be prepared for everything. Don't be shocked if you uncover them, and they find a way to get to safety.

Professional liars are easy-going who are able to make a deal through almost any circumstance. It's likely to be difficult to expose them with a lie that they aren't able to escape from.

A Sure-Fire Trick to Tell If Someone Is Lying

Here's a clever trick that you can employ to determine whether someone is lying. It's so effective that you could be enticed to solely rely on this method. Do not give into temptation. Learn to be an intelligent lie detector and make this a part of your weapons. This shouldn't be the sole weapon.

If you're convinced that you're being deceived about something, you can ask several questions regarding the subject and observe the person you're speaking to begin to shake. Each question must require an answer that is more specific than the previous. The longer the subject has to think about how to answer the question and the more they think about it, the more difficult. If the person is using a substantial portion of their brain to come up an answer it's more likely that they'll show body language that indicates lying. They're putting their brains to work for an answer that is reasonable, and it's hard to keep control of their actions.

You should wait until the subject really begins to squirm or become angry Then, abruptly switch the topic to something totally unrelated. A good example of this could be changing the subject from infidelity to the film preview that you watched yesterday. In reality, it does not matter what you change it to , as long as it's not related to the issue that you're discussing and is that isn't important.

The way in which the subject reacts will tell you whether they're lying or not.

A person who is innocent will be confused by the sudden shift in subject. They'll either speak about their confusion in a way or be able to seeably disoriented. It will take about a minute or two to adjust their minds to the new subject and they might try to discuss the subject again. The sudden shift in topic is stressful for the brain, and people will want to revisit the topic you had been discussing to conclude the conversation.

Someone who's guilty is likely to appear happy with the shift in the subject. Instead of becoming confused by the sudden change in pace, they'll feel happy that they're no longer being pressured until they're straining their brains to think of up a variety of lies. They'll dive into the topic without even blinking an eye.

This technique can be employed effectively to give you an idea of whether someone is lying or not. Be careful not to overuse it or your acquaintances and friends will think that you're an odd person who doesn't remain on the right track.

Another Sneaky Lie-Detecting Tactic

There's a second trick you can employ. This trick can overload one's brain with the lie-teller and causes them to struggle to think of an answer.

If you suspect someone of fabricating a story or fabricated story, ask them to recount the story in complete detail from beginning to final. If the story is long filled with detail and you're not concerned they know you're trying to uncover the act of lying, it might be beneficial to note down the specifics.

Ask them to start from the conclusion of the story, and tell the story by reverse chronology. They should provide all the information they had originally given. Someone who is honest can tell the story from beginning to the end, or from the beginning to the end without difficulty. The story is extracted from their memory and it isn't a matter of the order they recount it in.

Someone who is engaged in a lie has to fabricate the lie they're telling. They'll have trouble telling the tale in reverse, since their brains are operating at full speed trying to keep the story in the sequence they told it. Reversing the story can be too much for the brain to manage. It's possible that they'll mess up the sequence or stop for a long time while they construct the story in reverse the order.

Don't allow them to get away by merely stating the major details. You should expect the same level of detail that they provide when describing the story in chronological order. Be aware of them slipping through their sentences and try to piece it all together.

Be aware of their body and body language. The signs of deceit will be more likely be seen that they're offering the tale in reverse since they're experiencing a hard to put things together. There's no way to have the ability to control their actions when they are trying to reverse the narrative.

How to Expose a Lie

There are some who might feel content knowing you're being deceived by. If you're in that category, you don't need to read this part of your book. However If you're looking to expose a lying person in the eyes of others, then you're going be required to read this chapter carefully.

There are numerous ways to expose the truth. Beware that there are those who continue to lieeven after being they are caught with a red flag.

Pathological lying liars are so convincing with their lies that they've made themselves believe them. You can show an alleged pathological lie a picture of them engaged in the act they're debunking and they'll tell you that someone has manipulated to make them appear in the picture. If you show them a video, they'll claim it's not they, but someone else who appears to be them. You can catch them doing it and they'll later deny it.

They'll never admit to lying , and they create an complex web of lies to support their claims. The best thing you can do to do with this type of person is reveal them to wider world. If exposed, they'll be able to move on to a different group of people can manipulate and deceive.

If you're looking to expose someone for lying You'll need to do some investigation. It's not wise to go around asking every person that you can about the individual who you're concerned about as you don't want to be relayed to them informing them that you doubt the truth of what they're telling you. Ideally, you'd like to find a little information from time to time that will confirm your suspicions but without signalling any suspicions regarding your motives.

After you've conducted a bit of research, it's now time to engage in a confrontation. The trick is to conceal it so it doesn't appear like a fight. In a confrontational manner can cause the person to stop speaking. If you can, show interest in what they're telling you while asking them questions to find out more. They'll soon realize the ruse you've employed But hopefully by that point it's too late.

When confronting a suspected lying person, there are a few aspects you must be aware of. If you're looking to expose them to your personal information and don't worry about making them available to other people, you'll be more likely to gain more of a person by speaking with them in a one-on-one conversation.

The problem is that it's the other way around should you decide to reveal them to the public in the future. Don't believe that since someone confessed that something in front of you they'll be the same to admit it to the rest of us.

If you want to expose a lying person in the eyes of the public, you're likely require at minimum one reliable witness. Your BFF (best friend for ever) will not be considered an authentic witness. The person who lies will instantly highlight the fact that the witness is your closest friend and will support you regardless of what. It's now back to being their word against yours. A reliable witness is someone who does not have anything to gain or lose in repeating what has been stated or performed.

Okay. You're now ready to go. You're now ready to show this deceitful liar to the fake. One of the most effective ways to expose a deceitful person is to request for them to supply you with a an exact chronology of things that happened during the period that you are unsure of. If someone tells you tales of an untrue-to-the-letter vacation ask them to reveal what order they took things within.

If they say it was a day at the beach. They did kite sailing, snorkelingand then came across a gorgeous girl whom they went out with for dance and dinner after returning to the beach hut take note of the manner in which the things they did. Then, after a few minutes, bring the conversation back to the specific day. Change a few topics: "That sounds like an incredible day. Let me be clear you did snorkeling, and then kite sailing and met a gorgeous girl at the beach. After that, you went out dancing, went out for dinner before returning to your house? It was an amazing day."

What did we do? We altered the sequence of events by swapping dancing and dinner along with the kite and snorkeling. The reaction of this swap will give you an indication as to whether the tale is real or not. If someone corrects your mistake it's likely they're telling the truth. Or, they're an extremely clever lie-teller. A lie-maker who's not good at it won't be able to remember the order of events, and will instead be a liar.

Finding the order of events is a different goal. It permits you to construct a chronology of events. It allows you to analyze the order in which events occurred in order to find out whether there was enough time to allow for events to take place.

When you're determining the order of events, be aware of "logic gap." If someone is lying, they are likely to miss important details or give more information than required. Ask questions about anything that doesn't seem to appear to be logical and watch for any more holes to show up. The more lies someone must fabricate the more likely the story will become confused.

You should let the person you think lies do the majority of the talking. Ask questions here are in place to ensure that things are headed in the right direction. However, for as long as you hear someone talking about something, let them talk. The more they talk with their mouths and talk, the more likely to fall into the wrong spot.

You won't gain anything from your conversation. You're trying to gather information, not demonstrate your ability to speak in a way that you can be described as eloquent. A majority of lying people speak and even talk about the topic which they're lying about. They believe that the more detail they are able to give the more likely to believe the story they tell you.

If there were other people involved, ask them the way they participated. Find out specific dates and times. This will let you speak to others to determine whether their accounts are similar to those you've heard from your suspected lying liar. More sources that you've got to draw from, the more likely you'll be to discover an insecure connection.

If you're not able to debunk the deceit the first time note down your findings and do an additional amount of study. You can now probe and speak with witnesses who are relevant. After you've completed an additional round of research and have a good idea of the situation, you should return to the place of origin and ask them a second time. Make sure you have evidence to prove they're lying. You're trying to force the perpetrators into an alleyway, and then keep them there.

When you are asked an issue, be prepared for responses such as "I do not believe in theft" or "Cheating is against my beliefs." This kind of answer could suggest a guiltful conscience. It's time to seek the most direct response to your query.

Be sure to listen for phrases such as "to remain honest to yourself" as well as "truthfully." This means that the person is trying to convince you to believe the words they're using. People who are innocent don't employ these words often since they believe they'll be accepted as truth.

The person who has created an idea will stop when they are asked an question. The pause allows them to think of an acceptable response. They could try to hide the pause by yawning or a sigh, or they may request for you for a repeat question. In the event that you are asked a straight-forward inquiry and then the individual you're speaking to is asking what you're talking about you're likely to be stalling for some time. Time they'll use to come up with a lie.

Do not give the subject all the details you've got out of the gate. If you've got valuable information you can direct the conversation towards the information without divulging the details you have. Someone who is making up stories will not realize you already have the truth, and is more likely to make up stories about something that you know is untrue.

In the course of time you might be able to get some kind of confession. One of the most common tactics employed by lying liars across the globe when found guilty is to admit to something else than they're really accused of. A husband who says to his wife "OK Okay. You've got me. It was true that I sent her few emails, but I felt guilty, and I didn't get beyond the" is likely responsible for a lot more.

Do not fall for the first admission. Be persistent in seeking the truth until you are certain that you've made a complete confession. It's extremely uncommon for someone to offer up a full confession at the first time they make a mistake. This usually is done in the stages.

Types of Liars

There are many "liar kinds" that you can come across. It is helpful to identify the kind of liar you are dealing with when trying to determine if someone is lying or not.

Amateur Liar

This is the typical run-of-the-mill typical person who tells the truth. They do not lie often enough to become habitual however, they will sometimes lie to suit their needs. The majority of lies made by a liar who isn't professional are in fact white lies and aren't required to be exposed.

This kind of liar is easily spotted because they're not sufficiently trained to be able to conceal the signs they're lying. They exhibit body language that is a sign of lying, and they use speech patterns that reveal the truth about their lies.

Habitual Liar

The liar who is a habitual one is one who has a habit of lying. They are not shy about lying to reach their goals. They are more likely to lie at both at home and at work. People who are habitual liars usually lie for no reason. They're simply doing it because they are.

The most seasoned liars do not make a good job of concealing their actions. They make up so many lies that they're unable to keep on top of everything. They'll tell someone something, only to change their minds and give an entirely different story to another. Because they're known to make up stories about anything that comes to their mind and they're among the easiest types of liars to expose.

You can listen to various variants of the tale when speaking to a liar who is a regular. Speak to them and learn the tale, then wait for a week or two before bringing back the topic. It's likely that they've made up so many falsehoods, they'll never remember the lies they've have told you.

Pathological Liar

A pathological liar takes the habit of lying to a new level. The pathological liars are so adept in their lying that they can believe that they're telling lies that are real.

They often create crazy stories that seem absurd at first. A pathological liar can to present enough information and convey an account with sufficient conviction to make it seem convincing.

The pathological lie-tellers have no regrets regarding the lies they've told. If you share a story you'll hear one that's better than your own. They aren't happy to be overshadowed.

If you're dealing with a pathological lying liar you'll have to find small gaps in their tales and then dig into them until you discover the truth behind every lie. Don't expect a pathological lie-teller to admit to their mistakes. They'll keep stacking lies top of lies in an effort to get you confused.

Sociopath

Sociopaths are those who lie to make a name for themselves. They do not care about the opinions of other people and will crush any person who stands out of their path. They will lie to obtain what they want, and have made lying an art.

Sociopaths are generally more attractive than other kinds of liesters. They are loved by many and frequently have people eating out of their hands while filling their mouths with lies. I once met a person who told people that he had fallen over the Superdome as it was being constructed and that the only injury was a few missing front teeth. If you take a look the statement is clearly false. He was such a captivating storyteller, that nobody was able to doubt the truth of his story.

Sociopaths will be difficult to detect in a lie since they're typically adept enough to cover every aspect. You might be able to discern their facial expressions and patterns of speech sufficiently to be able to tell if they're lying, but finding them out requires some skill of your own.

The Professional

There are those who are so skilled in lying that it's almost impossible to determine if they're lying. They've been studying techniques of lying, and gone through the same books that those who spot lies have. They strive to be one step ahead of the most accurate lie detection devices.

A professional lie-teller will alter their body language to show they're lying. They'll also modify their speech so that everything appears to be in order.

The downside of a professional liars are the things they can't control. Although they can manage their body language to an degree, it's harder to control small details. Microexpressions are facial expressions that span the face for just a fraction of a moment before the professional can manage the expressions. It's difficult to detect the expressions, however they might be your sole possibility of identifying a lie in progress from professional.

Lying in Relationships

As the majority of our time is spent with loved ones than with other people, one might reasonably conclude that it will be easy to discern whether we're being deceived by the person we live with. This assumption is completely false. The truth is, we're much less likely to find our spouses lying in the event that they're not really lying.

The reason behind this is love is a desire to make sure they are the best of the person they've selected. We've all heard the expression "Love has no eyes." People who love each other don't like to think that they are being lied to by their spouse and often aren't willing to believe that they're being deceived to, even though all the facts are in front of them. The obvious fact to those being in the loop is ignored by the one who is being deceived by. It is a good thing to be ignorant in numerous relationships.

People like to give their loved ones the benefit of doubt. If there's a little doubt and that's what the person's heart is glued to. No matter how absurd the tale may seem the possibility is that it's real. They desire so much to believe in their loved ones that they're willing to ignore the factual evidence. The more deeply in love people are more likely will fall prey to this kind of thing.

It's not unusual couples to get stunned when they discover their lover in an untruth.

"I didn't know about what he was up to," they'll say. Truth is, the majority times, there were many warning indicators. The partner who was smitten decided to ignore them , believing they were not what they appeared to be like. This obfuscation of facts takes place at a subconscious level, and the person who did it doesn't even realize that they've done it until the actual event. Most of the time the warning signs aren't apparent when you look back.

To avoid this type of "love-blindness," you're going need to be very careful in examining the facts rather than thinking that everything is great. I'm constantly hearing people affirm that relationship are built by trust, and my suggestion indicates a lack in trust. My answer to this is to say that's what those who are oblivious to the warning signals say.

When you make a commitment to be part of a couple, the relationship must be an open book. You must have access to the e-mail accounts of your partner such as Facebook, Facebook, cell phone and so on. and they should also have access to your account. I'm not suggesting you swap passwords the moment you meet. What I'm suggesting is that when you decide to elevate this relationship further and transform it into an actual partnership and your relationship should be open to no secrets.

You're not alone You might be thinking, this isn't going to be a success. I discuss things with my buddies that I don't wish my spouse to be seeing. I'm sure he is the same way. Trust is a factor. Both of you have to make a commitment to not be upset about what you see in each other's accounts, in the event of a breach of trust.

There shouldn't be any secrets that are kept from one another. Consider it. If you're in a relationship today with someone who you've been in a relationship with for some time, and who has several accounts that you don't possess, aren't ever wondered what's inside the account? If you're in a bar with your significant other and they receive a message or two and they rush to reply to it, have you ever wondered the source of that text at a glance?

If you're not you're doing yourself a massive injustice. You're one of those "love-blind" people who later admit that they didn't know the truth behind their backs.

If you follow using the method of open books, you'll never be confused. No doubt. All you need to do is to ask, and you will be able to see who sent the message or log in and find out what your husband or wife is doing on Facebook.

Can this method totally eliminate fraud and lying? Yes, but those who cheat and lie create fake accounts and slyly go about their business.

What this method can accomplish is to reduce the chance of falling prey to temptation. There are women and men that have the habit of looking for people who are in relationships and attempting to lure them. Anyone who has an account that they only have access to is inclined to slip for this trap than one who's account is accessible to their partner.

Another method to keep an check on your relationship is to create a tight-knit group of people who share the same gender. Get together and discuss your relationships openly. You may have friends who are looking at something you're not. Don't assume that what they're saying is real However, don't dismiss the information either. If your friends say that the warning signs of deceit exist throughout your friendship, then it likely merits a second glance.

Examine the situation to be sure everything is upwards. The only thing that ignoring the issue can do will make you vulnerable to another major mistake later on.

I know a friend who was a victim of a man who took the woman off of her feet. She was a divorced single mother with two children. Although not particularly attractive, she was appealing enough to the point that she didn't have any trouble getting dates. She'd been seeing people for a while after the divorce, but wasn't in a relationship that was serious.

She ran into a man at an outdoor barbecue at the house of a friend. He was charming. He was tall, dark and beautiful--the entire nine yards. He was able to sweep his wife off her feet. He was loved by her Her kids loved him, her entire family loved him. He was too nice to be real.

There was just one issue. Prince Charming was known to be disappearing for days before he would return with a fascinating story about his being evicted at the spot for an "emergency" corporate meeting, or needed to rush away to assist an individual in need. When I mentioned to my friend that something was not right and she resisted the fact that something wasn't quite right.

"I'd be able to tell if the man did not lie to me,"" she added. "He's not a trustworthy liar."

She blindly believed in her boyfriend and didn't bother to look at the facts. I tried a few more attempts to persuade her to look at the facts and then gave up because I didn't want to lose my friend.

Mr. Perfect requested for her hand in marriage, and my friend agreed. They scheduled the date and created the arrangements. The girl I was with went to heaven.

Then it took place. A week prior to the wedding the bride's friend phoned me in complete hysterics. The husband she was about to marry had left his email account open and when she tried to shut it down, she saw some suspicious-looking e-mails. When she began to read the messages, she realized how blind she had been. Her fiancé had a lot of women he'd seen and even a few individuals she'd introduced him to. It's apparent that Prince Charming was charming everyone aroundhim, not only her.

The woman I spoke to was distraught. She later told me that the signs of warning were evident. She was too obsessed with love to recognize the warning signs.

Do not think for a second that this is an isolated incident. The same situation is seen repeatedly across all relationships. If you've been fooled to believe that you're in the "perfect" relation, the chances that you're deceiving yourself. If you're able detect the indicators of deceit you're far ahead of many.

People who are in relationships are often falsely confident of their ability to spot their spouse lying. They believe they've been together long enough to discern when they're fooled. Sometimes, they catch their partner in a tiny lie, and they think they'll be able to be able to catch all the lies. What they don't realise is that they're only getting only a tiny portion of the lies they're told.

Instead of digging further to find the surface of the iceberg They believe they're catching all. This leads to false confidence and lets them ignore the larger problems. It is important to keep in mind that for every lie you uncover in the first place, you'll find minimum ten times the amount of lies that are not being exposed.

I am in agreement that the foundation of relationships must be built upon trust. However, what I'm not happy about is the idea of building relationships on trust that is not based. If you find something that does not make sense or you're not sure about, investigate it more. It could save you some heartache further down the line.

Utilizing the strategies found in this book, you'll be able to dramatically increase the number of lies that you're getting caught and gain a good idea of how truthful your partner is to you.

That Lying Salesman

Salesmen get a bad rap. They're thought to be some of the most fraudulent creatures on the planet. Salesmen selling used cars are the most shady. It's a common belief that they'll offer you anything to make the sale.

My experience is that the trust that salespeople earn is very well-deserved. You'll encounter a few honest salespeople on the street. Similar to the way you can find an award-winning lottery ticket everywhere in the local convenience stores. There are lottery tickets however the odds of actually finding one are very slim.

Although most salespeople aren't taught to be honest but they're taught to conceal their information and try to scam you for every dollar you can put in your account. It's not that far from a leap for them to lie straight out to convince you to purchase products they can make the most profits from.

If you go to a location that has sales representatives present and not having all the information you can about the item you're considering buying is similar to cutting yourself and throwing yourself into the shark tank. If you are able to let the salesperson know that you didn't do your homework while letting the representative steer the discussion, you'll be creating a situation that will be disappointing as you arrive home and look at the "deal" that you just received.

In the past the only method to investigate an item was to visit showrooms or stores to find out what was offered. You'd be forced to endure sales pitch after sales pitch just to check out what was offered. If you're fortunate, you came across an incredible bargain on the product you were searching for. If not, you likely paid too much and came home without a clue.

The Internet is a wonderful thing. There is a wealth of information available on the Internet that lets you research the item you're purchasing as well as the most current prices and the best deals before even stepping foot into an actual shop. You'll have the information you require in order to be able to make an educated decision of the exact item you're looking for at a bargain cost.

I enjoy playing an unintentional game with salesmen I meet. It's known as "Play Dumb and See If They Try to rip You Off." I'll visit a store and ask questions about the item I'm interested in and look at what they are trying to explain about the item. I'm amazed by the number of salespeople are willing to completely be deceived to get a sale.

Here's a recent conversation that I met with a salesperson

I: "Hi, I'm interested in the Sony Vaio computer you have advertised for sale. It's for sale at 675 dollars. What do you know about it."

The salesperson listed several capabilities, some of which the computer did not have.

I: "Is it liquid-cooled? I'd really like to buy a computer that is liquid-cooled. I've heard they're better than air-cooled models."

Saleman: "I think this one is liquid-cooled. A majority of the new Vaio's are."

Me: "Really? I didn't even know about that. I was told by a friend that I should acquire a faster processor. Does Intel's Intel i3 a top of the best processor?"

Salesman "It definitely is. You can't get any quicker than this."

I: "Awesome, I was considering buying an Intel Core processor i7-3960X, and increasing its speed. What about that 3.3

GHx one? It's a lot more efficient than the i3, isn't it?"

The realization dawns on the salesperson who may have been trying to trick someone who is a little better about computer technology than he believed.

Me: "These computers aren't liquid-cooled is it?"

Salesperson: "Ummm, uh. I'm guessing not."

Salespeople start to get nervous as they realize they've in a tight spot. They're used to taking advantage of unaware consumers who have no notion that they're being swindled. When they meet somebody who is knowledgeable as or more about the goods they're selling and they are dishonest, it can make the honest one a little anxious.

A skilled salesperson will play with the cards. They'll be more than willing to discuss the item they're selling to them and appreciate that you've done your homework. If they're unsure of the answer you're looking for then they'll say they're not sure and discover it without fuss. A salesperson who is lying will create a story in a hurry, and then lie about the product to persuade customers to purchase it.

It's important to determine if the salesperson will be a fraud to sell immediately. I prefer to appear as if I'm not knowledgeable about products I'm interested in as it allows them the chance to make up stories. If they are lying about it, I'll move on to another place or call the company and request a different salesperson.

A common tactic used employed by salespeople selling cars is to offer you a reasonable price on the vehicle, and then push you to the curb in terms of extra warranty or financing. Be pre-approved for the loan online to give you an advantage in negotiations. Also get quotes on cars through The Internet the sales division of several dealerships. They'll be more likely to give you the best price.

When a salesperson claims to be telling you something so good it's impossible to believe It's probably. "This is among the best deals I've had the pleasure of getting from a client" actually means "I'm saying this since I've mentioned this to many customers in the past and it has been successful before."

If you're not sure whether a salesperson has been telling the truth, you can use your skills at detecting lies on them. Keep in mind that the indicators will be subtle since salespeople are taught how to make themselves appear more trustworthy. You'll have to be aware of what they aren't able to control, such as their pupils and their microexpressions.

Putting It All Together: Becoming a Human Lie Detector

Professionally trained individuals are able to detect lies with greater accuracy than those found through polygraph tests. The great thing about this is that you are able to detect lies at any time. It's not necessary to convince someone to permit them to be connected to a computer to determine whether they're truthful. You can connect them to your lying detector at any moment.

If you want to become a lie detector in the human race, you'll have learn to trust your intuition. If you're seeing multiple indications an individual is lying, odds are you're likely to be fooled.

When it comes to determining if that someone is lying, you'll need to search for "sentences" which indicate that someone is lying. One body language sign could be an accident. A whole set of indicators could be indicative of a deceit.

If you're speaking to someone and they've crossed their legs and arms and no other indications of deceit are visible The leg and arm crossed legs aren't a big deal. Perhaps they felt uncomfortable, or the conversation changed to a subject they didn't like or didn't want to discuss.

If you spot a signal that someone is engaging in a deceitful act and you suspect they are lying, take note of the other indicators displayed. If someone is bending their legs and arms then starts fidgeting and taps their feet to the ground is it time to listen attentively to the things they're saying and doing. Make sure you ask a direct one or two questions and watch for long pauses between responses or stammering and stuttering. Also, watch for eyes that turn towards the left or to the ground. If any of these indicators of lying are evident then you've now got an "sentence" of indications that someone is lying.

What you decide to do with the sentence is entirely up to you. It is possible to request more details to determine what the individual is doing. warning signs. If it appears that they're in a state of mind to break and you're willing to obtain an apology. The lies that aren't all important might be better left undiscovered. It's essential to recognize that nearly every person lies from time the other and there's no need to expose every lying. It's best to reserve your lying-exposing abilities for the more important issues. You won't have many friends if attempt to expose anyone who shows signs of lying.

The aim isn't to expose every falsehood that is presented. It's about being able discern the truth from the lies, so that you are aware when you're deceived by. The actions taken must be in line with the circumstances.

Chapter 8: Lie Detection

Lie Detection

"If you speak the truth you will be part of your past,

However, if you lie or make a false statement and it is exposed, it will be a part of your past."

The study of body language is called group study. This means that you should not be only relying on one gesture. it is better to choose gestures that belong to a particular category and then observe the gestures in the whole. Based on only one or two gestures be cautious regarding whether you are being deceived or lying about it. This could be a typical scenario where someone is frustrated, dislikes the person, doesn't feel sure of themselves, or is annoyed already. Therefore, it's essential to determine the base of the person's personality that is possible in the event that he or she behaves as normal. Check out how the person talks and laughs. Analyze the person's reaction and system, nervousness level or disorder, as well as emotional triggers. It's easy to get the baseline by discussing ordinary events, laughing and asking questions such as "How was your day Do not discuss directly what you'd like to discuss to avoid provoking the person. Liars can become aggressive when they encounter an expert in deceit, therefore do not judge a situation until you're in complete control. Otherwise, a routine scenario can turn into stressful when verbal abuse is used in response to the defensive nature. Fighting or fleeing is the normal reaction when faced with stress-inducing situations, such as getting caught, so a liar will do everything in order to succeed. In this scenario the brain doesn't have to be focused on the facts anymore. It is just trying to justify its decisions that involves assessment. It is the reason people try to justify their decisions as well as their thoughts, views and opinions or opinions, as well as critiques and decisions even though they could be incorrect from another's view. The mind creates excuses depending on the need and the ego. This is the reason I do not apply my research to any person, at least, not until I have enough control over the people and the circumstance. Nothing fazes me more quickly than someone who lies to me.

Every person has their own reasons and rationales. It is a fact that the brain prefers to reason rather than know the truth. 60% of people you meet are lying within the first 10 minutes. Based on of data collected, but the number of people who lie could be greater, and not lower. People can appear strange when they lie. It's because the brain controls behavior , and lying can put the brain into hyper-drive. It's a complicated task that stimulates the prefrontal cortex. This is the part of the brain that is which is involved in multitasking. If you are lying you are required to perform two things cognitively. In the first, you must block the automatic response that is coming from your body. This allows you to lie and tell the truth. Second you need to create the lie. Thus, your brain works more to fabricate lies than to reveal the truth.

It can be quite difficult to spot lies and requires concentration. The most significant issue is auto-suggestions from the mind and distractions. There's a lot to think about at the same time. The atmosphere, mood and mood, the topic of discussion, as well as the the seriousness of the event are the most important factors to keep in mind. Then will come additional sources such as tone, sound and volume expressions, words body movements, vocal and postures, gestures, sweating, flushing and so on. The verbal and non-verbal signals must be in sync. Because you are making a judgment on a person's intentions and character. This isn't an untruth! It's not required to believe that every information source is trustworthy and therefore determining the amount of deceit becomes difficult. Certain people are susceptible to leakage more than others , and certain people aren't. Some suffer from behavioral issues or character issues and other issues. It's challenging to keep both verbal and non-verbal behavior consistent when lying. The majority of people who lie cannot control their behavior when they are lying. They might not even be able to have the ability to control everything if they wanted thus it's possible that they leave clues to deceit. Be aware of the clues and be aware of what's concealed. A liar is extremely careful when it comes to words. His or her primary area of focus is focused on words, which means the reader's primary focus needs to be non-verbal signals, not the words. Do not be concerned if you miss some dialogues, but don't overlook any leaked facial or body signals. Every liar is a storyteller. What can you take in after all! The majority of people pay the attention to what's said. Though words are highly regarded, the majority of speech is not verbal. The new student can begin by watching body movements as it's difficult to detect the micro-expressions. The body can be a great source of deception leakage. Contrary to the voice or face and body movements, the majority of body movements aren't directly connected to the regions of the brain that are involved in emotions.

Shield Mode

The people trying to become secretive tend to cover their eyebrows-to-cheekbone area like a shield. This type of gesture is typically used to conceal a part of a facial expression the presence of a person, and to expose the face to another. It is a tactic students are taught to do in school where One side of the face, which is facing to the instructor is covered by the palm, while the other half is open to express their true emotions. The gestures can be seen unintentionally when someone tries to shield themselves while lying or concealing something.

The Mouth Shows it All

If you truly wish to succeed,

It is important to follow one rule "Never lie about yourself".

If a child is lying, his/her hands automatically move towards the mouth like the mouth is closed. As they grow older, this gesture gets more refined. It is presented to the mouth in a way that the truth is about to spill out, however it is difficult to stop the flow by using fingers and thumbs on the teeth and lips or using other objects. If people are prone to having opinionated or negative opinions about the person in the front of them, they use such gestures in order to express their opinions however, they are afraid of being judged; their body language does not cooperate, and they use the indignant gestures. If you're facing the person, ask them their thoughts but without getting defensive. Find out what they want to say. The truth will be revealed like it was dying however, a trigger prevented it from happening. Specific mouth zone gestures are commonly employed. If a person is able to rub his mustache (the direction that forms the French cut) from the philtrum up to the chin using his fingers and thumb indicates that the person is attempting to hide his deceitful thoughts or trying to prevent himself from being deceived.

Really Surprised!

If someone displays surprise over a long period for a period of time, that is the possibility of fake surprise or they are lying. The appearance of fake surprise is usually displayed by those who aren't afflicted with emotions as far as the subject is involved. If a person is aware of the truth but is amazed, an appearance of surprise and fake is created to convince people that they did not have any prior knowledge of it.

Itching, Isn't It?

When one person attempts to rub his back, it is suspicious and indicates that the person is trying to hide the truth. Itching is normal however, when someone lies then his or her hand will automatically rub the back of the eyes and cheeks, nose, the ear and face.

Time Travel

Expressions of joy, anger and other emotions are displayed just when the conversation is being conducted. If someone is faking emotions like hatred, anger or jokes, and the expressions occur following the words, the person is more likely to be lying. The real feelings of anger anxiety, and joy are evident through the flow of speech not just after the sentence has been said. The people who control and dominate others employ these tactics when trying to manage a situation. If the anger they express is real the words and actions will be in tandem or the situation could look like a instructor is trying to manage the students by using fake anger!

I Respect You

"People aren't interested in hearing the truth due to

They don't want to see their hopes to be destroyed".

Gentle and polite are morally required in our modern society. In the environment of Indian traditional family values it is considered impolite to express a negative tone at someone's face or engage in excessive eye contact with the elderly. People often present their personalities as friendly and agreeable when they are having a conversation, but their body language can be always negative. For example one might declare, "Yes I'm with you' however his head is showing "No, no way and moving between left and right and it could mean that they are lying. If he really is in agreement, the head must be pointing downwards, not to the side. A cooperative facial expression is essential to reach an agreement on something. many people use it to demonstrate fake respect. The fake respect is identified by observing the face. Chin thrusts are an indication of anger and disrespect. If someone continues to show chin thrusts, that's an indication of disrespect towards the person standing in the front of them.

Chin thrust

Blinking Beauty

The eye blinking rate is between 19.6-26. An rate of increase the rate or decrease it is an indication of danger. An increase in speed in blink rate can be used to detect a lie. A slow rate of blinks indicates that the person isn't paying to the situation. The eyes are irritated and blink more frequently, however a skilled person who is lying blinks less since professional liars train beforehand to detect the smallest signs of deceit. Being under investigation is an arduous task for any person. If, while being interrogated there is no indication of anxiety or stress or anxiety, they might be well-prepared as even a calm person experiences anxiety when dealing with investigators, police or any other.

Poker Face

In no other area does the body language research become more specific and weaker when it comes to prediction, however we require more specialized topics like microexpressions where the lie can last for just several milliseconds. A poker face is typically described as a face without expression that doesn't reveal anything: good or bad, sad or even happy. A face like this is generally neutral most of the time , and smiles could be fake. Poker pros who are successful are usually proficient at keeping their emotions under control, and employing the fake body language. This is why they choose to wear dark glasses, so that the pupil's reaction is unnoticed. Professional players with an understanding of deceit and body language, wear fake body language to fool others and make them feel confused psychologically.

Prepared Liar

A lying liar with a plan is very dangerous. It is important to observe the time it takes to respond to your questions. If the time to respond is shorter than the average time in stressful situations this could be a pre-planned lie. Anyone who is confident and a normal person, who isn't a threat, may become anxious and nervous when repeatedly asked questions can cause confusion in certain circumstances. It is therefore a cause of concern when someone appears confident enough and is able to respond with less than the normal time that is expected in these situations. In such instances the person asking the question should be calm and allow the person to be able to tell the story in his or her own method. If you are suddenly being asked to tell the story in reverse order from the beginning to the beginning, keep in mind that it's difficult to create a tale in the reverse direction. They will make mistakes with no knowledge of the proper sequence and the actual worry in the throat and eyes is easily discernible. The person will always look at the sky to create a visual representation of a fake story. This is enough...no further evidence is required to conclude that the individual is lying. It's best to threaten them so to ensure that truth come out.

No Money Hidden Here

"Listen and listen to the words of others. do Not say ..."

When someone hides an item such as money, drugs, or other items the person will feel anxious as well as warm and nervous when an inspector gets near the item. Their face will display an uneasy anxiety in their eyes, and anxiety at the back of the throat. To ensure this, move the spot around and watch the person. If they appear more relaxed and content shortly after the change It's a red alert. Choose the spot you like and begin seeking out what the suspect was hiding. If you're an investigator with CBI or Income Tax, this trick can be very effective. CBI as well as Income Tax this technique will be a boon. All you have to do is be able to play Hot and Cold with your opponent.

Messy Lipstick

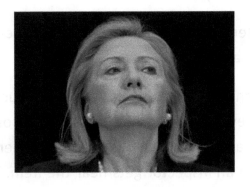

"Quiet People have Loudest Mind"

- Stephen Hawking

If someone ties their lips while speaking it indicates that the person in question has something in mind and is ready to reveal it, but chooses not to talk about it. It could be that it's not important or they don't want to reveal it! This characteristic is similar to lips that are pursed and is a variation of this. It's similar to when an individual applies lipstick and then meshes her lips to evenly distribute it evenly. If you see this kind of gesture while conducting an examination, it's a signal of concealing. Explore further to find out. If you are a normal person in a situation where you aren't able to use force or force, don't hesitate to take the initiative to change the body language defensive.

Oh My So-Called Well-Wishers

"Trust is just like an eraser. It becomes smaller

and then smaller for every error".

"Beware my"well-wisher!"" You will be saying when you learn about this feature. It explains that timing can be an essential tool when deciphering an untruth. If the timing is not in line with emotional expressions or words i.e. the difference of time between what is spoken and the emotion that is that is expressed e.g. for example, when a person who greets a bride and the groom at their reception by and saying, "I am very happy for you both" and smiles when she says that rather than at the exact moment when she said the statement and then smiles, she is fake.

Therefore, the timing and duration of emotional gestures and declarations should be done in accordance with a normal rate. The delay in emotional expressions is an indication of over-exaggeration. Sometimes, an emotion shows up and then disappears completely from an individual's face which indicates that the emotion's cause isn't as important to the person and the person is trying to make it appear more significant than it actually is.

Truth Behind a Truth

The most clever lie-tellers are often extremely smart and will do their best to divert your attention. When you begin to investigate them and conduct an interview, they'll attempt to alter the subject into details that relate to another fact regarding the topic. Imagine that you are looking into the kidnapping of a girl and having question-answer session with victim's friend's relatives and their close ones. One of them is in a state of anxiety and whenever you try to speak with her, she begins to tell an additional story about her, the man she was with, or even her the use of drugs. You'll believe it when it's true but it's also easy to cover up the truth behind a less important truth in order to escape the suspicious eyes of police. She will tell you the truth and you trust her! You can now be free from the real tension behind a more threatening truth.

When you're dealing with a clever lie-teller, be sure to remember your true subject and motive due to the ability of the suspect to hide the truth. Take note of facial expressions, even after the suspect has told you the truth. Act like you believe him/her. You will eventually see the anxious look which has become more relaxed, unless the suspect is able to distract you from the game.

Fingers Create Storms, My Dear

If someone is manipulating or lying, the way they move their fingers reveal a lot. Anyone who makes gestures with fingers such as pointing at someone frequently needs to perform gestures that are symmetrical with words. When making a statement, as and pointing the index finger upwards and then looking into their eyes and then look at the fingers. They should coincide in direction.

It's fine if their direction is the same, but when your finger is pointed in one direction and the eyes are directed in towards the other direction, it's a sign that the person is making up thoughts in the mind that does not believe to be factual. The mind is so busy to produce things that it is impossible for the body to keep up with it.

Like Me, If You Can

Hostility can be hard to identify when someone is attempting to appear it is difficult to tell. But, it can be identified by three signs when talking about someone that the suspect is averse to. If you are unsure about whether one female acquaintances doesn't enjoy a different female and you want to know why, ask her how she thinks of her. You can ask her to provide an introduction that explains what she is feeling. If she is able to touch her eyes, nose and lips' corners, and then smiles in a mocking manner by closing her eyes , and raising her lips to one side, then she's lying. The incredible things she has said about the woman is a lie since the presence of negative body signals in this instance is more than normal. How can people be sure of the truth? They boast of honey, but are not ready to hurt like bees. Humans are extremely complex. I've seen people have a lot of fun with one another and act as if they are friends, but actually quite jealous of each other. Be attentive to how someone speaks about someone else to you, because that is how they describe them to others.

Offensive vs Defensive

It is essential to recognize the distinction between being defensive and offensive. An innocent person can become defensive when confronted by a truth or lie, whereas the innocent can become offensive. They will be angry, which is also normal because of the sudden and unexpected blame. Imagine someone accidentally blaming you for ruining his vehicle the night before. At first, you'll be astonished (eyebrows raised and mouth open lower eyelids widening and horizontal wrinkles appearing across the forehead) then within a few seconds, your shock will change into anger. "How could he possibly say these things?" you will say in anger, becoming abrasive, furious and trying to get deeper to defend yourself, but your anger will be there until the very conclusion.

However, in the case of the second in which you have really damaged the car, you'll be surprised for longer than the normal amount of period of time. Your voice will be more nasal, and you'll get defensive and won't need to address additional details when it's being used against your. People who are self-conscious aren't willing to cooperate with truth-finding investigation However, it's difficult to discern the lies of those who believe in their own deceit. If this happens then they cannot be labelled as liars because they do not show the signs of deceit. This is why the psycho is very confident when he tells lies, and those who suffer from self-doubt are unable to see the full reality. They are masterful liars since they don't feel any guilt. Their mental state is influenced by their false convictions.

Have you met anyone who is deemed irritating and, whenever asked for advice,, behaves outrageously, making sarcastic remarks and fun ways to laugh off your worries? Someone like this shows that the question you asked isn't to be taken seriously. He/she even makes jokes about you, which can lower your confidence. This is the most convenient method of hiding beneath the cover of 'laughing'. Beware of someone who laughs at questions and responds in a way that is irrelevant to the questions you ask. They discourage you to not ask further questions. Avoid these individuals, but if you must deal with them, you must have the authority to confront them and be able to keep your dignity and respectability to manage the situation together with your partner.

Reverse Politics

Public speakers are extremely, excellent in deceiving. They train a lot prior to speaking in public, and over time, they have accumulated decades of knowledge, they do not need to do any practice before putting on the disguise of deceit before the public. Politians, who are the most lying people, know a good amount about deceit and body language. They also know about facial reading. They know that experts are watching them everywhere they go, so they do their best to reveal any signs. In general, they think of their lies, or do it before mirrors or with hired experts such as script writers. In such instances there are a few ways to decipher their lies. One is to be aware of microexpressions that will be explained in depth lateron, and the other is backward-speaking. Instruct them to speak their stories and plans backwards. They'll forget or not remember the story because it was done only in one manner.

Fear of Being Caught

Human beings are part of the world where each person's survival depends on the cooperative efforts by all members. This is the main reason why people make up lies. The loss of credibility can happen after being discovered by an extremely high-risk lying. The truth can cause the death of our honor to our social system. There is no one who will cooperate with those who are known to have been involved in serious lies or crimes, adultery and fraud. In Indian society relationships are the basis and the basis of marriage, business as well as social interactions are based on honesty as well as co-operation. Honesty is among the best traits that people seek in their loved ones, friends or partner, a relative and leader , and the repercussions of a breach of trust are threatening. Family rejection is the main fear of those living here. For the same reason, people are known to lie about matters that are of various magnitude. They are able to lie in both negative and positive situations. From the beginning of childhood, Indians are good liars because of the high-voltage reaction and the expectations of their elders. Evolutionary history hasn't taught anyone to be adept at detecting lies However, Indians are masterful at lying. They may be aware of every ritual and habit of a family member , but they are unable to comprehend what is going on inside the brain of that individual. In India the average wife will spend about half a century together with her husband and isn't able to see the true picture of her husband's thoughts because of the lies they've told one another over the years. To be a great lie-teller, one doesn't have to be two-faced which means they display one face to the public and at work, and the other face to family and friends. The third one they keep to themselves and not for the sake of a show! It's a bit complicated isn't it? This is the harsh truth. Today's generation is looking for change and are fighting religious and social taboos as well as fake reputations that are based on falsehoods and old convictions. They will surely have to be subject to more criticism and disdain and continue to fight to make a changes. Independence and honesty are the top priorities of our generation. With the many opportunities available technological advancement, industrialization, and the massive power of the young it is not as many negative social consequences like previously. Privacy is easy to obtain. It is possible to change the spouse, job, or where they reside (from city to village). A bad reputation does not have to remain with his way. This reduces the risk of the harm that lying could cause. Technology, like cameras and mobile technology can deter us from lying. If caught, it's easy to find and gather evidence of the crime using the location of the crime, camera footage as well as other technical records. Only a few highly experienced criminals can escape from these crimes.

Backing up the Truth

"Don't be a believer in the stories of people who claim to say they will

Secrets of other people's"

People who typically begin sentences with words like "to be honest" or 'truly', be honest and honest and honest' and "let me reveal the truth' are a regular liar. Why is it necessary to use the term 'true often if you are speaking the truth? Is truth so paralyzed by the need for additional support prior to speaking? People often require these phrases before speaking because they don't trust their own words and they believe that they aren't able to promote their conversations without adding words. I've often heard these phrases in conversations and find it difficult to sympathize with people who aren't confident in their own words. There is a lot of usage of these phrases on television, specifically by actors, politicians and news panelists, where they repeat things they do not believe in accordance with their scripts! It's enough to speak. They pretend that everything before these words is a lie, and that everything that follows will be a lie too.

The Power of Mathematics

This is known as the game of numbers. If you wish to confuse your suspect and gain more clues of deceit and truth, you can enthral the suspect with numbers such as "how many", "how much"', "AM/PM Rupees' and other numerical questions. In the case of numbers, confusion can decrease the confidence of your suspect because he'll need more time and attention to respond before speaking. Puzzles can loosen his grip on body language and expressions to the point that the truth will be revealed out naturally since the art of understanding form and not all people are artists.

Scrub Your Temples

A forehead that is smacked while speaking to anyone or working in a group can be a sign of confusion and confusion. If you are in an exam hall, you'll notice many candidates making this gesture because of uncertainty when answering. But smacking and hiding the nose in an examination may be an indication of deceit and fraud. Take particular care, watch those who feel itching in the nose. It is difficult to tell if they are cheating or talking to people in the room with them.

You are Staring Now

It is a well-known fact that people do not make eye contact when lying, however according to research smart liars have more eye contact in order to gain the certainty that you will believe their words and lies. Nowadays, people are experts thanks to television, education as well as the web. We are constantly bombarded with information, and confidence is their mode to live, no matter how many lies they have to tell.

Many jobs today are based on lying and people are prone to lying. They don't believe it's a crime, and they don't feel shame and it's much more difficult to spot lying people these days since they don't defend themselves and don't make eye contact. A lack of shame has diminished the importance of truth since people are incredibly comfortable with lying. They don't feel ashamed when confronted with truth, unless of course you're a police officer! If you're a family member or friend, liars may be defensive and aggressive because they believe they didn't do anything wrong.

Looking Daggers

A frown usually signifies displeasure. The way we look at our eyebrows is to convey anger, displeasure and mood swings, which is a common expression employed by children and women. The timing and its relevance to the message is crucial when detecting the deception. The absence of any relevance from the words is a contradiction to the message. If a woman tells a man "I truly am in love with you" but in contrast she smiles and smiles, an untrue message is being communicated. The signals she communicates verbally and non-verbally are in opposition to one another.

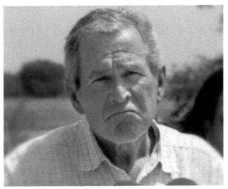

Because the Mouth Comes Up With a Lie

It is the mouth that is final communication device for lies and can tell us something about the lie-teller. Mouth shrugs are among the most common gestures of slip that indicate the lack of faith in the words spoken! It resembles the half pout, where the corners of the lips are directed downwards with forceful mouth movements. When faced with stressful situations the mouth shrug signifies the feeling of helplessness. Watch any video of celebrities talking about how the upcoming film can inspire and change in their lives If this gesture is used repeatedly to convey a message, it is likely that the person is lying and is trying to draw attention to the "movie on sale". Also, when you view videos of politicians on the campaign trail as well as TV hosts and businessmen, you'll see a lot of these gestures. This is a sign of doubt or a lack of confidence, as they don't trust what they've said It is recommended to think about it before deciding. Let's take the instance of a businessman speaking about his future plans commitments, plans, and his business before the media, and asking for people to put their money into. A continual shrug of the head indicates that he's not telling the truth or isn't prepared to take a huge step in business, to the extent that he talks about to the general public.

Mouth shrug, example

Memories Warm up the Head Inside

The process of interrogation can be a challenge for any person. The pressure to provide a satisfactory answer to an inquiry creates the specter of deceit. When a question is posed in the absence of any past experience or guilt connected to the question, we can respond just 'yes or no', 'ok or 'I don't have any idea as short responses. However, when there is a memory connected to the question or answered, the person who gives the answer is more likely to defend themselves by citing examples, excuses of global beliefs systems as well as clarifications. For example I asked my friend if she was a backbiter , and she replied by saying 'No, I don't I don't remember that I did', her thoughts contradicting the facts. Perhaps she had a memory of the latest incident of backbiting, and tried for me to prove as many as she could to prove that she would never ever do that. "Oh you're right Don't believe reports," she would say. Of of course, someone who never ever backbites may also offer the same answer. that's why window dressing necessary? Simple is the best. We're human in the end! We all gossip and backbite It's more likely that she has never did it. Although window dressing phrases are often used by people who use emotional blackmail and thugs, they might take the questioning too seriously, as if you've offended them. If I asked my aunt the exact same question, she'd reply, "Can I ever do this to you! You are aware of how ashamed I feel when I say these things about my beloved ones. I'm unable to even hear this kind of conversation, so how do I say such things? I'm against it." That is a clear and obvious act of deceit. To make it sound more genuine the liar gives abstract assurance of innocence through personalizing and universalizing morality. The reason for this lies in the belief systems which requires an additional source of support to make up for the deceit. They often continue to talk until they get your response because their brain hasn't reached the level of trust that is required to trust them.

I'm Not Really a Liar

There are a variety of methods to spot lies, but in certain circumstances, people alter without the intent to lie. They are frightened when they feel anxiety, fear, or sexual arousal too. It is essential to determine how these emotions affect women and men before making judgements about anyone. The face may turn red in the face of the desire to be awed, shy, or anger, not just guilt. Therefore, a variety of microexpressions and body language are essential and a mutual knowledge of the comfort level of the individual must be present before the rules are applied to the prospective.

The worry of getting caught is a good thing in dealing with suspects as it assists in leaking non-verbal clues. The suspect needs to believe his lies will be discovered. Fear signals are the subject of debate. The liar is the only one and not the truth-teller is afraid in this kind of circumstances. We must remember that self-confidence diminishes the capability of deception to detect terror. Criminals, conmen and stubborn people can make use of the power of their confidence. If they believe they can escape you can!

Yes or No

Words should be in agreement to body language. If someone says yes, but their head says NO i.e. that he's not indicating a nod but is turning his head to the side like the person who said no which means the person isn't confirming his assertion. The heart and the mind are saying"NO" but his body language declares YES. In the school there were students who could never complete their assignments and, when they saw their teacher, they would always say, "YES ma'am, I will be done by the next day, sure," but their head was turned in a different direction, which meant no, don't even think about it!

The same is true for other gestures. Our gestures should confirm what we're saying. Eyes should be looking in the same direction where our hands are pointed. It's a lack of connection between mind and words; it indicates that the mind is not in sync when we speak.

Glamorous Indian Weddings

In the event that you imagine Indian weddings, what you think of is a glittering, crowded place that is filled with glowing, smiling faces of both genders who have fun and laugh with one another. There's also a ton of food, laughter dancing, drama, and joy. This is the only location where couples' families can enjoy all the time they can and enjoy a very hard-earned celebration. Even the middle-class have a wedding of a grand scale in India that even the top middle class can't pay for in western countries. In India, the Indian wedding is the way that each family from India showcases their. Who says that Indians are easy to get along with? Take a look at the wedding below and you will see that nothing is easy. It's a long-lasting wedding celebration, where each element is crucial and without the need for compromise. But, but, wait.... This is the flip side of the coin. perhaps a little odd or offensive... But the truth can be said to mean that Indian weddings can be described as a massive auditorium full of lies, masks shame, embarrassment, embarrassment anger, jealousy as well as personal satisfaction, contempt as well as a display of many other emotions together in one place. These smiles are a good indicator of the things they truly wish to convey. I am awestruck by the sight of people tell lies and making up stories about every aspect. Sometimes I doubt and laugh at myself and wonder what would happen if all the world learned to tell lies and using body language? Weddings would cease to be celebrated in this manner and only a handful of people who care deeply about the brideand groom and their families would be left. The rest of the people familiar to us, such as our family members, are who are part of the group. This is a crowd of regular people from India who know our identity.

Too Much Sugar

If a story is created out of a story, at least one or two items are usually not included in it. Events that are invented are singular in nature; they do not contain any negative information. The person telling the truth would have positive and negative emotions that were experienced, such as 'the train was late', 'I'm overwhelmed and exhausted after the event' and 'the event went off well'. Someone who lies will hide the actual basis of the story and will give you the positive claims made up by the person, such as "The food was fantastic" she was fantastic the night before The date went well', 'I was satisfied and motivated every day the show went with a flourish', etc. There is a normal tendency to anticipate positive and negative events when something really did happen. This theory can be helpful only when the event occurred in recent time and you're asking for immediate details since the mind tends to forget the smallest negative details within a few days, unless something very negative happened. It is common for us to want to keep the memories happy and positive so our brain immediately erases any negative aspects.

Why Everyone Lies

If you're in an incident where everyone in the people are lying begin talking to one individual however, observe the facial expressions of those around them. If they do not display any emotion or agree with the assertions made by one of the speakers, could all be lying or trying to conceal the truth. The absence of emotion is equally crucial in certain circumstances and so is the presence of emotions. Imagine you are investigating the aftermath of a sexual assault at work where the victim is able to describe what occurred to her. It's natural , however when they don't show any emotion, it's best to check everything again and comprehend the reason behind this lack of emotion.

Fed Up of Your Lies

Signals that lie, such as scratching your nose, closing the ears and touching the collar closing the mouth, or scratching your eyes when listening can be a sign of displeasure for those who listen. The various gestures you make during listening mean that you are aware they are lying, and fake it on a regular basis and you're totally annoyed by their lying. The mind cannot accept that they are lies. That's the reason it attempts to block the sound bits they tell you from getting to their ears. The person listening says in his head, "Stop liar, enough of your lies. Stop talking to yourself."

Verbal clues allow us to identify deceit while confronting the liar. Verbal hesitations, such as the over use of 'oh "ah," "hmm," and 'err' in sentences; repetition, changes in the form of statements and slipping of the tongue indicate that there are a few shady conversations going on but it is important to distinguish these situations from boredom as these signals indicate the degree of interest a person has and whether or not he is keen to speak to you. A significant rise or drop in the tone of voice similar to that of the stock market curve indicates the presence of anxiety. Are there any reasons to be concerned?

Bobblehead Liar

A lying person is not comfortable in front of the person asking questions, so he'll attempt to move his body and head away. If he is in the presence of others, he'll be able to make assertions and glance at the person in front of him and nod to ensure that at the very least, the other person is convinced. This is the best method to deter the questionerthrough using another person to use as weapon. If you're a lying person do a little making a nod in front of a man to build his trust. If you do, the person asking the question is likely to lose confidence and motivation to go on for any length of time. This is usually the case when confronting questioners at work or with family members and friends. A lie-teller tries to win the other person's attention in order to increase confidence, and also weaken the person who is asking the question. Therefore, it is best to be a solo speaker in case you truly want to control over the lie-teller. You can make use of your weapon against him by attracting attention to another. Investigators from the police usually ask questions in three groups in order to intimidate the suspect. The suspect is unable to believe when a group tries to intimidate the suspect and there is no way to cover up the fact that he is being investigated. An emotional weakness triggers a person to burst into tears.

Biased Judgment

If you already love or dislike someone and it affects your judgement. If someone's problems are similar to yours it's possible to subconsciously influence your opinion. You're not likely to fall for these tricks, however, the most common bias is the belief that you are impartial.

There is no such thing as a natural lying. People tend to develop into liars because of anxiety, peer pressure or a tendency to show off and many other factors. It's difficult to discern between an uninvolved's fear that they will be believed and the guilty party's suspicion. The purpose is to identify the lie-teller, not for a person who is innocent to commit a crime he hasn't done! It is not our intention to discredit a lying person because of his confidence and talent in attracting people. Be aware that your judgement should not be based on appearances, appearances or creed, color and race. If your thoughts still influence your decisions due to these factors it is important to be aware of your biases and avoid making any rash decisions. The responsibility of a behavior analyst is far greater than you could imagine, since trust is the most difficult thing to acquire, yet the it is the easiest to lose. You shouldn't violate the trust of those who trust that you. When I first started reading faces and acquiring how to speak, and was quick to express my opinion. I became and stayed friends, despite having certain non-believers. My father encouraged me to limit my actions of giving opinions in a flash if not requested. My predictions were like an athletic game with a ratio of 75:25. It was enough to get me noticed but I later realized I was not right to make predictions and make comments about people based on a lack of knowledge and skewed opinions. Then, I made the decision to build my knowledge enough to be able to express my opinion and perspective. I remained silent and in control throughout those years of basemaking. It was difficult to maintain my control knowing the thoughts that were going through the minds of those who couldn't talk due to fear of being rejected and the fear of being judged within themselves. It's offensive, and difficult to label the person who lies lying. Therefore, it is better to remain still and concentrate on your business when your advice is not being asked.

Policemen and detectives, as well as special agents must strive to be aware of their own prejudices regarding the person they are investigating. Because of their constant interactions with suspects, criminals, as well as terrorists, the behavior tends to be more suspicious of other people and consequently they have a lower tolerance to individuals. The normal behaviours that are exhibited by suspects could be perceived as deceitful by the suspects. When dealing with a parents, children, or spouse who has shattered trust the people who work on the subject of lying detection may be tolerant and make the fatal mistake of denying the facts. The mistake of believing that deceit is unjustifiable. False perceptions about people can hurt their reputation or make someone fearful to commit the crime they hasn't committed. The aim is to identify the lies and not to terrorize innocents. Anyone who works in this field need to recognize that they are victimized by their own assumptions to the point that they are unable to be sure whether or not someone is lying.

Active/Passive

"Tell a lie and all your truths

become questionable."

They are comfortable making passive statements instead of active statements. Making direct statements is an emotional pleasure for their psyches. They are able to add words into their conversations instead of uttering "raw lies" because they can show their expression of fear and anxiety. They don't want to share unnecessary details because of this.

If you discover that you have been deceived Should you take action against the lying person immediately? Do not do it! Continue to talk in a normal manner. Take advantage of the conversation since it's entertaining to hear lies once you are aware of the truth. The best strategy is to maintain the peace that exists between you. This is the way that you can avoid having more lies revealed as you continue to talk of conversations. If this happens the suspect will become anxious and cautious. So continue to gather evidence and truth before you seriously ask the suspect questions.

OMG! Why a Pause?

Voice is a major factor in determining the truth of deceit. The pauses in voice are among the most obvious indicators of deceit. A long pause and frequent pauses in conversations could raise suspicion. The lie-teller will try to fill in the gaps to increase confidence, but there is always something that appears awkward and unfinished like the pauses are creating an echo. In these instances the possibility of detection is high. could cause the liar not remember his lines due to the fear of being detected. In the case of voice the most reliable indication of emotion is pitch. The pitch increases when the person is unhappy. When sadness is caused through fear, the voice that is angry is high pitched. In situations of extreme nervousness and fear the voice/pitch begins shaking like the person in question is about to weep. The fluctuation in the pitch - high-low-quickcan cause anxiety in the speaker's brain.

The liars do not like the pauses and silences in conversations. They attempt to fill in the gap by using silly words or defend them. Laughter is among the best methods to make up an illusion; the quantity of laughter that occurs in conversations is a sign of the degree of trust between the two speakers. A lot of laughter or fake laughter suggests that you're making use of laughter to cover up the weaknesses in your argument. It's the most common indication of deceit. A fake smile is only for a few minutes. If it ceases, a part of the smile is lost and real laughter can bring a smile to the face, even after laughing. If you are laughing too much is, however can be an indication of a inattention and lack of communication.

Changes Causing Satisfaction

If you've come to the conclusion that the individual lies, change the subject of the conversation swiftly and demonstrate that you are completed with prior conversations. The person who is lying follows the conversation and is more relaxed when he uses less defensive body language that was previously a hindrance. The person who is guilty wants to change the conversation. The facial expressions have become more comfortable and calm and the eyes appear more normal, the expression serene and content. It could be the result of a tiny expression of unidirectional anger that shows the ability to conceal the truth with aplomb. A person who is innocent might be confused by a sudden shift in the subject and might need to return to the topic of the prior. The facial and body movements of an innocent person seem more shocked and relaxed than someone who is guilty.

Many people feel guilty lying, however lying can be enjoyable for a lot of people. It can be seen as a success, which is a good feeling. The results of a lie which succeeds is viewed as a reward for the lying liar. The lie-teller feels joy and excitement, as well as satisfaction, pride at the accomplishment and disdain towards the victim. The people who cheat don't do it at random They commit the crime by decision. Keep in mind any time you had a conversation between your friends, especially when jokes are made in the form of faking a friend's identity for amusement. A smug smile is a natural thing to see in these fun-filled moments. The pride increases when the prank succeeds.

The guilt of deceit is greatly influenced by the fashions, culture as well as peer pressure. Although ragging is considered to be being a crime under legal terms enforcement, it continues to be practiced with a variety of ways that remain hidden. Students are required to confess their ragging experience in order to express their joy in having rubbed one over. Seniors are happy when they share their ragging experience of juniors. A lot of the ragging performed to those who are ragging indicates an authority.

Red Working Alert

The act of lying is an extremely unpleasant experience; it decreases our effectiveness and makes it difficult to perform the task with the same level of effectiveness. One cannot work at the same level of effectiveness and speed that could have if he's been lying or concealing something. A decrease in efficiency at work is also possible when a person feels ashamed but isn't showing emotion. After being freed from this guilt, they will be caught back the same way. Increased speed is possible in the case of anger, but a lack of expression our feelings. The output quality could be affected due to rough handling however, the speed is quick. This is the same when we're satisfied, but with the added advantage of high-quality!

The cause of this shift has been uncovered by scientists who conducted numerous experiments to uncover the truth behind lies. Neuroscientists have observed that the brain performs more when it's lying in comparison to when speaking the truth. Researchers discovered that just four brain parts were activated during telling the truth, whereas seven were active when lying. The difference in brain state can make it difficult to complete other tasks when lying. A sudden drop in performance is evident, particularly when we're concealing something or are lying. Remember when your mom could detect something wrong by looking at your academics, sports or your routine?

Scientific Explanation of Touching the Body

While Lying

Entrepreneur

The nose Erectile tissues in our noses that increase in blood volume when we lie down. It causes a tingling or itching sensation, which requires the use of a nose to relieve it. A lack of nose contact does not mean that it is true, however, having a touch on the nose often is a sign of deceit. Of of course! There are times when a person may touch the nose due to cold, but with a bit of training, you can recognize a fake nose contact from something innocent.

Speech problems when you lie to yourself, cause our brain to think that the lie is true and that the reality is false, and at the same time, we remember that the actual truth lies within each other. Are you confused? The act of deceit can affect our ability to think efficiently. When we lie, we are more prone to pause and speak slower than we normally do and have speech problems which serve as fillers for gaps such as "uummm," "err," or 'hmmmm. Learn to recognize the deceit when you hear this type of cue in the form of a verbal.

Incongruous behavior - If our body language and words aren't in harmony the communication we are making is not in sync. Imagine you ask the salesperson if he could ensure that your order will be punctual. If he explains how certain the delivery would be punctual while turning his head from right to left (no) then he's not in agreement. If this type of incongruity occurs, you'd do well to put your faith in the body and not his words.

Neck rule: We rub our necks as a result of the pressure we feel when we think the challenge is unsolvable. Imagine you're interviewing potential employees for a job in the leadership field and the potential candidate expresses his enthusiasm in the job , but starts with a neck rub as the duties expected of him are described. It's likely that they don't believe that they will be able to fulfill those obligations. It's possible that he's wrong because of anxiety, but if there is anything we know about the human mind, it's this the case: if someone believes they're capable of or cannot accomplish something, they are likely to be right!

Interviews

Hiring and interviewing employees is among the most important jobs in any business, no matter how small or large. People with talent can alter the fortunes of a business. The business's mission statement is based entirely on the employees as they are the ones who bring it to life. The process of hiring isn't easy since it's normal for a candidate to lie about himself in order to be hired. The most effective way to get an interview is to lie! The applicants try to portray their qualities in a positive appearance, which leads to many lies being told. They try everything they can to hide their negative points and exaggerate their positive points, however there is an upper limit to everything and a distinct difference between fraud and window dressing. The word "fraud" is not justification for a lie to falsify documents, identity documents, police verification, past experiences as well as old and recurrent scandals or suspensions that are connected to the candidate are totally inadmissible. There are several ways to are able to lie about their resumes during interviews:

1. Refuting to reveal family history

2. Falsely stating the date of employment

3. Inflating numbers and percentages

4. Making up degrees and lying about them

5. Paying higher than the previous one.

6. Titles that are inflated

7. Acquiring fluency in a variety of languages

8. Making up technical skills and experience

9. Giving false personal information

These statements are often based on falsehoods, but there are some that are acceptable for a skilled and competent job. Personal issues pertaining to someone's private life may be overlooked but not educational or professional requirements. It's difficult to believe that more than 70% of former applicants admitted to having admitted to having lied during their interview.

Lie Detection: Visually Remembered and

Visually Created

Eyeballs move automatically in various directions when talking between left-right and up-down, each direction having a particular significance. When a right-handed person attempts to recall something that actually exists, their eyes will automatically shift towards the left. It's a visual memory. an opposite to visual creation. If the eyeballs are moving upwards to the left, it's possible that the person is inventing something The majority often an untruth. Naturally, this expression could be tested with youngsters. You can ask them to remember or talk about their most recent experiences in the outdoors. You will observe that their eyes shift toward the left. After listening to their thrilling stories, the other children of the child will get enthusiastic too and will try to relate their experiences, even but nothing has happened that deserves attention. This is why they to lie. They glance to the right, while constructing falsehoods.

Visual things that are routinely seen are easy to recall. When you require you visual memory recall specific images, you'll glance to your left e.g. What was the most lively and sly within your classroom? Your eyes were moved to the left to remember who was actually there however, when you are calculating the visual constructs, your eye is moved toward the right. What would a rose look like when it was black with white spots? What would your mother look like with hair that was blonde? To picture these images the mind automatically guides your eyes to the right.

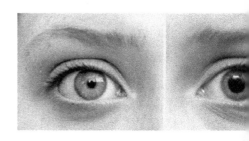

Remembered Left

Created Right

Troubling Smiles

"Beauty is power, a smile is its weapon."

- John Ray

Smiles are the most commonly used mask to disguise other emotions. It decreases the chance of detecting deceit. The expression of any emotion can be altered by using smiles to deter a person's attention at just the right time, and especially when it appears natural. If you're too fast or slow, an expression that doesn't alteration in the eye area appears unnatural and forced. What I'm trying to affirm is that it's much easier to fake a smile whenever circumstances require it since it's the very first expression we have of our origin. To fake such negative emotions as sadness/stress/frustration is more difficult than smiling because it is hard to convince the mind to act stressed when we are happy/normal. We are all aware that lying people are like they are deceiving. They do their best to hide their faces but it's very difficult to keep voices, words faces, feet and hands in tune. If you have a few hours of practice watching people, you can quickly determine if someone is fake stress or sadness.

Early methods for detecting a lie

Ford (2006) said an article in which one of the earliest methods used to verify the authenticity of a claim made by an accused documented in China about 1000 BC. The person accused of lying was asked to fill up his or her mouth with a small amount of rice. After a few minutes, the suspect was instructed to vomit out the rice. If the rice was dry, the person was found to be guilty of fraud. The method was built on the principle of physiological chemistry and the belief that the experience of anxiety and fear is often caused by a decrease in saliva and dry mouth. The writings of modern author (Matsumoto and Prasko, 2009 Prasko 2011,) suggest that fear can paralyze us physically and manifests by an increase in heart rate, as well as a feeling of hopelessness. The physical manifestations of fear and anxiety include changes in behavior that are accompanied by the sensation of dry mouth. The cause is comparable to the symptoms of panic disorder, depression and similar disorders (Hoschl, Libiger, & Svestka 2004). Due to the fact that the above-mentioned knowledge of the physical signs of anxiety weren't available at the time and therefore was not taken into consideration and the vast most prisoners irrespective of whether they done something wrong or had lied or not, were executed. Some years further on Erasistratus, Greek physicist and doctor (300-250 B.C.) was attempting to spot fraud by measuring the pulse. The same technique was used again as part of the polygraph testing in 1921 (Trovillo 1939).

The trial-by-ordeal method

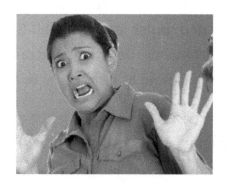

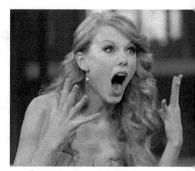

The writings of the past from various European nations more frequently mention the practice of trial by ordeal which is also known as Judgments of the Lord (Apfel 2001; Holak, 1974; Sullivan 2001). Another method was used by authorities with the aim of deciphering lies and finding the truth. It was used to establish the credibility of claims of an accused by an exact act that the accused must go through. Based on the favorable or negative outcome the claim was accepted as either true or false.

The reasoning (and consequently arguments of courts) was built on the belief that God will not let an innocent man suffer or let injustice rule. For instance, in the present-day territory of Slovakia early courts had been set up around the year 1111. They were either a one-sided confirmation of truth made by an accused or a double-sided one, in which one was judged of God (Holak 1974). The one-sided judgement of God was accomplished through either a water or fire test. The test of water was performed making use of cold or hot water. In the case of the hot water test, the person accused was required to place his hand into a pot of boiling water, and then remain for a specific period of duration. If the hand immersed in boiling water was not showing any evidence of blisters or scalding that could be a proof of the accuser's assertion to be correct. Another variation of this test required the suspect removing stones or a ring from the cauldron filled with boiling water.

The test, based on cold water involved throwing the person in the water with a rope bag. If the person who was tested emerged from the water within an insignificant amount of time was a sign it was a sign that "not even water will accept the person" or more specifically"servants of the devil" (hence the word "liar" too) refused baptism, and that is the reason why water is unable to accept them (Sullivan 2001, page. 213,).

Concerning this method of hot water there were some who doubted the validity of this method. In 1593 In the Netherlands the court referred to a school and asked for an examination of the test of water to assess its validity as a method of detecting lies. In this instance, reason prevailed which led to the testing being deemed unconstitutional

(Apfel 2008). However, the test using cold water was popular up to the 18th century, as shown by court records from Vojtka along the Danube where 70 women were subjected the test (Holak 1974).).

When making use of fire in a proof method, the suspect was forced by a heat source to transport a piece metal for a specific distance, or walk on the burning embers. The accused was judged innocent if there were no injuries were visible or they healed rapidly.

Sometimes , the court resorted to the practice of a consecrated meals. The person who was being examined was a priest who after the service and apologizing to the accused, handed him the bread and a slice of sheep's cheese that was hard. The accused was honored when he or she was able to swallow the whole thing without difficulties. If, however, the individual suffered a choking or death during the test, it resulted in an indictment of guilt. There are some similarities between this test as well as those of Chinese practice of using rice. In China and in Europe the population tried to discern lies by employing the mouth. However the Chinese method of verification relied on the fact that they had a good understanding of the signs of fear in the body - when fear is present, the mouth is dry.

Methods based on God's decision were no longer in use after the 15th century and only the test of cold water mentioned earlier was left. It was used mostly to verify witchcraft. The public began to realize that the innocence or guilt of an individual was not able to be determined by different "experiments" that relied on supernatural forces or gods that had the ability to safeguard innocent. The shift in perception of truth and deceit came with the gradual development of different fields of science.

Phrenology and graphology

The year was 1870. Franz Joseph Gall discovered an entirely new method of detecting deceit by the being able to detect the emotions of the suspect. The idea was further developed and improved upon in cooperation with his pupil , Spurzheim. The focus of their research was the study of certain regions of the brain and that there are connections between various abilities and the skull shapes (Rafter 2005). The principal concepts of their theory pointed towards the brain as being the principal brain organ that can detect individual emotions like aggression, emulousness and destructiveness, and, among numerous others, the tendency to deceive and engage in criminal behaviour. The most active areas of the brain can be identified from the contours that the brain has (these regions were more concave or convex). It was thought that the size of each of these areas could be increased or diminished through training and self-control. Gall was a pioneer in studying the skull of the human being and the newly-founded scientific field was called Phrenology. Gall frequently appeared in public in which he displayed criminals' shaving heads, and also emphasized their "anomaly" on skulls. By using phrenology, he attempted to identify liars by randomly selecting from the crowd. The services he provided were often employed in legal proceedings to determine who was lying.

Within the field of criminalology Phrenology was instrumental in spreading the idea that criminal behavior (together along with lies) ought to have a place in research. It bolstered the medical model of criminal behavior based on which the actions of certain criminals could affect their brain dysfunctions. Because of this theory the severity of crimes was reassessed, and prevented a variety of mentally ill individuals from being unfairly punished (Trovillo 1939). While phrenology was largely forgotten and was dismissed and discredited, Gall's work provided an important contribution by reminding scientists of the fact that human bodies are influenced by external factors, and they form an organism of mutual relationships (Hall and Lindzey, 2002).

Alongside phrenology, the term graphology started to gain popularity and by 1875 began to be considered a viable scientific method of detecting lies (Schonfeld 2007). The origins of graphology are linked to the attempt to identify fake signatures that led to science-based analysis we see it today. Its creator, J. H. Michon believed that certain characteristics of handwriting might be linked to specific characteristics of a person's personality. Based on the study of handwriting, graphology tries to determine a person's writing pattern that reveals the personality of the writer can be revealed (Schonfeld 2007). The fascination with graphology as a technique for lying detection was waned after the First World War. The wartime use of graphology was seen as a valid method to verify authenticity of papers as well as signatures. However, it was not recognized as a reliable method for detecting lies. In the present, this method is utilized in many fields like employment profiling (to create a profile of a person's personality) as well as psychological analyses (used in conjunction with other assessment tools for projective personality), (Poizner, 2012; Thomas, 2001).

Contemporary Methods of Lie Detection

The polygraph

In 1881, following the discovery of phrenology the first modern device for detecting lies known as Lombrosso's Glove was developed by an Italian doctor, criminologist and Anthropologist Cesare Lombrosso. He tried to determine the changes in a suspect's blood pressure that were then documented on charts or graphs. The sophisticated technology was further developed throughout the First World War by William M. Marston and developed into the final version following the war in 1921. The device could be used to track variations in blood pressure as well as breathing changes as well as give evidence (Trovillo 1939). The device was later used by John Larson and Leonard Keele created a psychiatric device dubbed "Cardio-Pneumo Psychograph" often referred to as a polygraph, or a lie detector (Lewis and Cuppari, 2009). The polygraph measured respiratory rate as well as blood pressure variations as well as changes in galvanic skin responses (bioelectric skin reactivity). Based on the fact that research studies (Lewis and Cuppari 2009) highlight the relationship between diaphragmatic and thoracic breathing as an indicator of emotional stress and changes (male and female breath patterns in these signs typically differ) modern polygraphs can examine the rate of breathing in the abdomen and chest separately. This results in a significant improvement in the diagnostic significance of the measurement. The foundation for assessing the results of a test is the relation between changes in physiological function that occur when someone does not tell the truth. The changes can be measured and observed through the use of a polygraph, which includes skin conductance blood pressure, breathing rate and heart rate. However, the changes in your body may vary, and can be caused by other states than lying (Brewer and Williams 2005). In this type of testing two kinds of tests were tested namely those of the Control Questions Test (CQT) and the Guilty Knowledge Test (GKT). The most common polygraph is the CQT because it is frequently utilized in criminal investigation. The CQT usually asks suspects two kinds of questions: control questions as well as relevant questions. The control questions relate to the suspect's criminal investigation, but are not specific to the criminal act. The test tests the extent to which the suspect is aware of a crime the suspect does not wish to divulge. For instance, a examiner of the polygraph might talk to the suspect a variety of kinds of cars and one was utilized in the commission of the crime (Lewis and Cuppari 2009).

In the latter half of 1990 in the late 1990's, the polygraph was beginning to be utilized throughout the United States not only by the police , but as a way to verify the credibility of public safety workers as well as managers (verifying the authenticity of information they provided in their CV, previous jobs as well as other information.). Because of its increasing popularity and frequent, false results the reliability test was carried out on polygraph. National Academies of Science (NAS) declared the polygraph's reliability as 81%-91 percent (National Research Council Committee to Review the Scientific Evidence on the Polygraph 2003, page. 4.). The results were confirmed by research scientists like Fiedler, Schmid, and Stahl (2002), Bartol and Bartol

(2004), Grubin and Madsen (2005), Grubin (2008), Lewis and Cuppari (2009), Ginton (2013). For instance, the symptoms of anxiety, nervousness and emotional disorders are seen not just in those who report false information however, they also occur in those who are honest. In the end, it can be said that the polygraph doesn't detect deceit, but instead it detects physiological responses that have been suggested as being related to deceit. These responses are not specifically associated with deceit or are all the time present when deceit happens. But, when utilized by trained examiners when used in conjunction with other methods it can be an effective method of identifying people who are trying to trick (National Research Council Committee to Review the Scientific Evidence on the Polygraph 2003, 7). 7.).

Examination of nonverbal gestures and Voice Stress Analysis of nonverbal expressions and Voice Stress. The need to identify lies isn't just evident through the use of different technological devices. Attention and observation focused on specific facial expressions can also play a significant role. Darwin (2002/1872) explained Duchenne's work in 1862 that suggests that we can discover the truth through the observation the facial movements. A smile that originates from happiness manifests itself through contraction of the zygomatic major muscles (musculus Zygomaticus Major) which causes the teeth's corners to raise. When there is an the muscle being stimulated electrically it is not natural. Similar to the circular muscles of the eye (orbicularis Oculi) that, when tightened will pull the face a little higher and raise the eyebrows. These two muscles may reveal the real state of your emotions as their activities is controlled with great difficulty, as noted by Charles Darwin in 1872 (Ford 2006).

In the 1960s, Ekman initiated a series of cross-cultural studies that focused on expressions of the face emotion, gestures and facial expressions. Alongside his fundamental research into emotions and their expressions and expression, he was also researching deceit. In the year 1991, Ekman carried out a study which he studied the ability to spot the lies of people from various occupations. The study focused on specific jobs where people have to confront the most often with lies. Participants included members of secret services psychiatrists, judges police officers, people who operate polygraphs and university students. Participants were required to explain the shifts in behavior and facial expressions and the voice intonation of the woman who was giving evidence and, using these clues, arrive at the conclusion that the testimony was authentic or not. The most effective group of participants was shown to be that made up of agents from the secret services. The authors saw a connection of this conclusion due to the fact that the majority of them had experience in the protection of prominent state officials, wherein at public events they were required to rely on the non-verbal reactions of those who were in the crowd. A negative correlation between age and performance was observed by observing that people older than 40 years of age had higher scores. Researchers believed that junior colleagues had more expertise in their field, while seniors tend to be more working in the administrative field. Kohnken's study (1987 and cited in Vybiral 2003) regarding the investigators' ages revealed negative results. Through instruction of police officers the positive correlation of age with the success in detecting false eyewitnesses was discovered. Senior investigators were more successful in detection. Additional results from Ekman's research provide evidence of the lack of performance of psychiatrists and judges in detecting lying. Judges' inability to detect lies was explained by the fact that they cannot observe the face of the witness, as witnesses often are in a place where judges cannot observe the person's face. Judges are more likely to concentrate the attention of their listeners, and making notes. Psychologists did not think it was crucial to identify the lies at first, as they believed the lies would eventually surface up to surface (Ekman and O'Sullivan 1991). When interpreting the findings is a matter of taking into account that the mentioned research focused mainly on the possibility to provide a credible delivery of emotional states (videotaped nurses) as well as the related type of lies that conceal emotions, which could greatly impact the likelihood of generalizing the results. Ekman pointed out the differences between what people believe and what they are aware of. This distinction is attributed to the fact that many people overestimate their abilities to discern falsehoods (McNeill 1998).

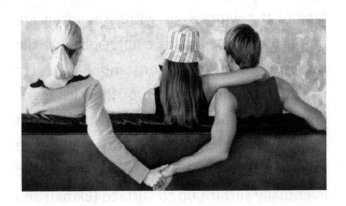

Craig, Hyde, and Patric (1991) conducted research that helped clinicians recognize distortions in the experience of pain which include a deliberate attempt to minimize the display of pain (masking) or over-exaggeration of such behavior (simulating). The authors identified facial movements related to masking and simulating as well being genuine pain. In response to this research, Galin and Thorn (1993) conducted research that concentrated on the detection of fake expressions of pain with the aid of the method known as FACS (Facial Action Coding System). FACS is a tool for research which can be used to determine every facial expression that humans can create. FACS is an anatomy-based method for describing in detail every facial movement that can be observed. The method was developed by Ekman in 1979. The method was later upgraded and named Ekman Micro Expression Training Tool. The instruction manual for this technique was made as self-based instruction. In other words, users would study the guide, take a test using video images then take an exam to be certified (Ekman 2015).

Furthermore, Ekman (1996) presented six theories on why we're not succeeding in detecting lies. One of the main reasons is the evolution of mechanisms for authentic disguise as well as the detection of deceit. Communities were always close together , and had few options to cover up cheating. Moreover as was noted at the beginning of this article, the revelation of lies can lead to the use of harsh punishments. Conditions of living have changed dramatically and the society offers more opportunities for lying. In some instances, even encouraging its citizens to lie or even to employ lies that are not true (e.g. advertising sector and trade, as well as business). However, we have the ability to recognize falsehoods (Vybiral 2003). According to Ekman (1996) tends to be predisposed to trust , which can make life easier. For the fourth reason, Ekman (1996) mentions the fear of being fooled or to not know the truth. This includes situations where we don't wish to be aware of certain facts, and therefore aren't able to make inquiries (e.g. when with relationships). One of the explanations by Ekman are based upon the findings of Goffman (1974 in Ekman, 1996) in Ekman 1996) who says it is crucial to be accepted by society as well as affable and not tell the truth (so-called"courtesy lies"). The final explanation is directly related to those who specialize in detecting lying. We have observed in the study by Ekman (1996) however, none of these studies demonstrated the ability to detect lies. In this situation, the suitable method has been shown to be training using FACS (Facial Action Coding System) which allows successful detection of lies through the examination of emotional expressions in 70percent of the cases (Matsumoto, Hwang, Skinner and Frank in 2011).

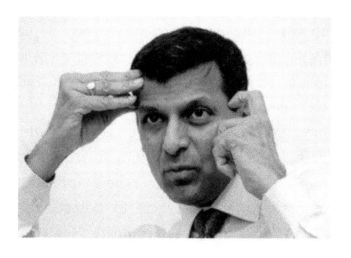

The expression of emotional states is a result of another method known as Voice

Stress Analysis (VSA). The process of analyzing voice stress (VSA) is achieved by monitoring the changes in the physiological micro tremors that occur in the speech. Micro tremors are low-amplitude oscillation of the reflex mechanism that regulates the tension and length of a muscle due to the finite time delay in transmission between neurons and from the muscle being targeted. Microtremors are found throughout the body, including vocal chords. They are characterized by a frequency of 8-12 Hz. In times of stress, the microtremor changes in frequency. This shift in frequency is transferred from the muscles of the vocal tract and into the vocal. Based on these results it is believed that the VSA is believed to be an effective method to, for instance, to detect false claims. In a study that compares the two, Patil, Nayak, and Saxena (2013) declare that the frequency of micro tremors in Voice Stress Analysis (VSA) technology is able to detect emotional stress more effectively than the polygraph. Patil et al. (2013) proposes a further tests of the reliability of the VSA for identifying false statements in the realm of justice.

Brain-based lie detection

In the years between the 1980's and the advent of neuroscience, completely divergent opinions about whether it is possible to determine what what lies at the very top level of brain activity have been uncovered by means of analyzing brain activity, like transcranial magnet stimulation - TMS, magnetic resonance imaging (fMRI) and positron emission tomography PET, and Brain Fingerprinting (EEG wave). As of the time of writing, research papers related to this topic are being published by Bles as well as Haynes (2008), Ganis, Kosslyn, Stose, Thompson, and Yurgelun-Todd (2003), Langleben et and. (2002), Lee et al. (2002) and Spence and others. (2001). In this article, we discuss the most commonly used techniques that include Brain Fingerprinting

PET, EEG and fMRI. Guevin (2002) explained the very first method for Brain Fingerprinting developed by Donchin and his student Farwell in the year 1990. Brain Fingerprinting is a way of detecting a specific EEG (electroencephalograph) wave. The hypothesis suggests that brains process certain and relevant information in a different way than how it process irrelevant or unknowable information (Farwell and Donchin 1991). It is believed that the brain's process of processing certain information, like the details of a criminal's case stored in the brain is revealed by a particular pattern that is detected in the EEG (Farwell 1994; Farwell & Smith, 2001). Farwell's fingerprinting of the brain initially used the well-known P300 brain signal to determine the brain's recognition of well-known information (Farwell 1995; Farwell & Donchin, 1986 1991). Later, Farwell discovered the P300-MERMER ("Memory and Encoding Related Multifaceted Electroencephalographic Response"), which includes the P300 and additional features and is reported to provide a higher level of accuracy and statistical confidence than the P300 alone (Farwell, 1994; Farwell, 1995; Farwell, 2012; Farwell & Smith, 2001). In peer-reviewed research, Farwell and colleagues report less than 1% errors for laboratory research (Farwell and Donchin 1991, Farwell & Richardson, 2006) and in field applications that are real-life (Farwell Smith and Farwell 2001; Farwell, 2012). In an independent study, Iacono (1997, as referenced as cited in Allen & Iacono, 1997) confirmed Farwell's findings (Allen and Iacono 1997). In spite of these results that the brain fingerprinting does have some limitations. In order for these methods to be useful in the identification of crimes the researchers need to have sufficient details about the incident and the person who committed it. This is required to determine an individual suspect's EEG patterns once the right response is given. It is also possible given the ferocity of the media's coverage that suspects could have details about an offense without being the culprit. Brain Fingerprinting is expensive and requires more preparation and time than a typical polygraph this, together with the patent granted to Farwell limitation, has limited the range of how this technique is able to be utilized.

Other options for using graphic brain imaging technique for purposes of lie detection include functional magnetic resonance imaging (fMRI - functional magnetic resonance imaging) and the positron emission tomography (PET) which concentrate on the activities within the central nervous systems (brain and the spinal cord) and not the peripheral nervous system (neurons). In another study, Langleben et al. (2002) utilized BOLD (blood oxygenation level dependent) FMRI to try to pinpoint the changes in neuronal activity of the region when deceiving.

CPSIA information can be obtained
at www.ICGtesting.com
Printed in the USA
BVHW042325150223
658636BV00021B/312

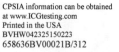

9 781998 901524